LIGHTNING BUGS

the iceberg of mental illness

by

Mike Lima

Dorrance Publishing Co
585 Alpha Drive
Suite 103
Pittsburgh, PA 15238
Visit our website at *www.dorrancebookstore.com*

ISBN: 979-8-88925-459-1
eISBN: 979-8-88925-959-6

"All actions are lessons, everyone you encounter is a teacher and your entire life is your education."

-Mike Lima

This book is dedicated to those teachers, my wife, children, grandchildren and my great grand daughter who died at two months of age. Thank you all.

Chapter

1

When I was eight years old, I convinced a friend that I had gone to military school and I knew how to fly an airplane. We decided to take a trip. Actually, we decided to run away from home for some reason or other. We were going to go to my great uncle Donovan's in Withie, Wisconsin. I had been there last year and thought it was cool, and it was the only place we could think of.

I grew up in Galesburg, Illinois. We lived at 534 Monroe Street, next door to a city cop. Oscar Babbitt was a grand ole man, friendly and very kind. If I remember right, Oscar played the sousaphone in the police band.

It was 1955 and the Municipal Airport was located at the southeast corner of Fremont Street and Highway 150. That puts it close to a mile away from my house. It was a long walk, but that was the plan. Walking is nothing for a kid.

Jimmie Gaines, the friend I had chosen to run away with, and I walked to the airfield and looked around. The airplane hangars were close to Fremont Street and kind of lined up along Henderson. We pushed open a hangar door and there was our plane, a yellow Piper Cub. It is a very light aircraft, so we pushed it out of the hangar with ease.

I got inside. I had watched pilots start airplanes several times on TV shows. However, they were the kind where someone had to stand in front of the plane and give the propeller one or two spins. The guy inside, me, had to operate the controls, give it the gas, and engage the brakes and… everything else.

I told Jimmie to stand out in front of the plane near the engine and propeller as I had seen them do on TV. He did his part like he knew what he was doing.

I did not have a clue in the world what the hell had to be done first or for that matter, what all really needed to be done. I only knew if I could get it going, I could fly it. I just knew that I could fly.

Bad news, I had to admit to Jimmie that I didn't know shit. So, I told him that this was a different kind of plane than I was used to flying at the army school.

The first signs of problems surfaced while attending L.T. Stone Elementary School. During recess in first grade, I picked up some rocks and broke the windows of my classroom. I don't know why, I just did it. Then at a P.T.A. meeting, I left the gym where Mom was attending. I went to the second floor of the school and set off the fire alarm. That caused quite a commotion. They did not catch the culprit (me).

In second grade, I was bullied. There were these two cousins; one of them lived across the street from me and I thought he was my friend.

People have told me I get this look in my eyes and it scares them. I guess I had the look that day. I lit out running toward these two jackasses and they took off. I chased them for about three blocks, and they ran into Ronnie's house. The next day, a Galesburg Police Officer came to school, pulled me out of class, talked to me, took me home, and talked to my mom. The parents of both cousins had called the cops on me when it had been their two brats being the bullies and causing ME grief.

It was also in the second grade that the kid living over on Henderson and Grove and I had found a bunch of pop bottles at an abandoned building at the same location. We grabbed a case each, went into the middle of the Henderson Street (Hwy #150), threw them into the air, only to break in the middle of the street. Why?

I sure as hell have no idea. I figured I was just a bad kid. A State cop saw us. He made us clean up the mess, and took us both home and talked with our parents about it. No charges filed.

My brother was four years older. One day, he did something to me that really pissed me off and I got that look! He took off running, I chased him around the house, then he ran in the front door and locked it. I started beating on the door's glass. I put my fist right through it. Mom took me to the emergency room. I had to have seven stitches in my hand and four in my finger. There was blood all over our front porch. Everyone was more scared than I was.

In the third grade, there was a bigger bully. A fifth grader. He was pushing and shoving me all the time. Up to this point, Dad had always said, "No cussing and no fighting." That all changed after I came home crying every night after school.

Dad said, "You have to fight back." I told him this kid was big and Dad said, "Then you have to get an equalizer." I didn't understand, so he said, "You have to get a rock or stick… something to even the odds."

So, the very next day this kid was pushing me harder. I saw this brick laying on the ground. I picked it up and I threw it on his foot. He started crying after he fell to the ground. He left me alone after that, though.

His parents called the school blaming me because he broke a toe or something. I was on the "hot seat" again.

The school psychologist talked with my parents and recommended I get counseling. Dad would not hear of it. He was 'old school.' Boys will be boys.

Leave it alone. Besides, his son 'could not' have mental issues. Yea! No counseling for me!

back at the airport

What a letdown, but Jimmie bought the story I made up about not being familiar with this type of plane. We walked the mile back home, only this time, for me, it felt like a three or four mile forced march. It was my walk of shame and I deserved it too. I was such a big liar.

I watched lightning bugs every night during the summer. They were my friends and the closest I was going to get with my flying for a while.

The 'lightning bugs,' (along with Sky King) were part of my dream for wanting to be a pilot in the first place. They took off and flew around with ease. They flashed their light just like the rotating beacon on an airplane, so every other 'bug' could see where they were and where they were going. It was all so simple.

That's the way I saw it, in my mind. Simple. So easy. I never let that dream leave me. Ever! I already knew how to fly. I was born to it.

I think my mom knew it too, but she never let on. I knew that she knew, because she was always buying me books about aviation. She also was aware that I was spending all my allowance on balsa wood airplanes and cherry cokes at Nelson's grocery store down on the corner of Monroe and North.

I went to that airport almost every day and watched the planes. Taking off, landing, doing touch and goes, and just flying. In my mind, I was in every plane I saw, and I was either the pilot or the co-pilot. Then, in the summer of 1957, it all was coming to an end. We moved about ten miles away, to Oneida, Illinois. That did not change the plans in my head.

It did complicate my visits to the airfield. Although my days at the airport were limited, I was still a pilot. Sometimes I would ride my bike to Galesburg and go to the airport. Sometimes I would hitch a ride or go with Mom and have her drop me off for a couple hours at the field.

Many of the pilots noticed me hanging around. They knew my name and I learned some of theirs.

I always thought Mr. Currie was the owner of the airport. He was, in fact, only the Fixed Base Operator. He managed the field and had certain privileges. He was also the Chief Pilot and had the plane rental agreement. The city of Galesburg owned the airport. Mr. Currie lived just down the street from our house, on the corner of Grove and Jefferson. One street over from Monroe.

So, every once in a while, Currie or someone else would take me up and show me the ropes. I was a quick learner and even got to take the controls sometimes. I was having the time of my life and it kept me out of trouble. That was an extra. It was really good for me, having this dream.

Chapter

2

It had not occurred to me that World War II was over. My driving ambition was to be a fighter pilot in that war. My dad was in the Ploesti oil field raids in Romania. Their B-24 Liberator was shot down along with many other planes on the raid. After they bailed out, Dad landed, straddling a fence.

One foot was going north, and the other foot was going south. Ouch. His ankle was broken. Consequently, the Germans never 'set' it properly and it had to be re-broken when he came home after the war. Holy shit! Double ouch!

He was listed Missing in Action for some time, and then Mom received a telegram from the Department of Army. It said that he had been taken as a Prisoner of War and was in a prison camp in Bulgaria.

Mom already had some information about that from Dad's grandmother. Grandma Ward was very religious, and she told Mom that the Lord had shown Harold to her in a vision. He was alive, but there was something wrong with his leg. Sure as can be, that was the case! Grandma told Mom this long before the Army telegram had ever arrived.

Dad came home in 1945 at the end of the war. He was on crutches. If he hadn't made it, I would not be writing this. So, this would be 'no more' than 'just a dream.' I was born in 1947. My ideas about flying entered my head about six or seven, and it had just not registered that I was too late for getting into the mix of WWII.

When I finally did put it all together, it placed a damper on me for a while, but it never rattled my dreams of being involved in aviation. Up into the wild blue yonder I would go, just like the fireflies, someday. I'd never "give up!"

Sky King and Penny were still on TV and the "Songbird" was still in the air. With each new year, the plane was a newer model. And every year that passed by, there was a new version of me too. I was not a kid anymore, I was growing up! Boy, I was really getting old! I think I was eleven or twelve when it hit me about the end of the war. I still refused to believe it. Eventually, it sank in.

I started the fourth grade in Oneida. It was a rough start. I was trying to make friends, so I told them I was a professional baseball player. They believed I was on a 'farm team' for the Chicago Cubs (what a whopper). Worse yet, I was no good at sports. They all learned that when I failed to 'stand out' at a recess ball game. My lies had put me in another predicament.

I kept telling stories though. However, I learned to alter them so that they weren't about me, but just funny stories they would like. I had become a successful actor/comedian. It was all going well. For now, anyway.

I was also still up to no good. I took my cousin in tow. We went to the local tractor dealers. I knew this from our tractor. Back then, there were no keys, just an ignition switch. If I had known this fact a few years ago, maybe I could have gotten that Piper Cub started.

These were all used tractors. We would borrow any one we wanted and drive around town for a while, then return it to the holding yard. We were lucky nothing ever went wrong, and we never got caught.

Another really stupid thing I convinced my cousin to do was try smoking. Most kids try this sooner or later, but our escapade was dangerous. We went to the grain elevator, hid in a room and lit up.

We had NO idea just how explosive grain dust is. A simple spark can light it off, and here we were lighting matches to smoke. Grain dust explosions can blow up a whole city block and worse. We were both great-grandkids of

Grandma Ward. I think her prayers were protecting us. At least we had a mention with the Lord!

Then disaster struck again in sixth and seventh grade: cars and girls entered the radar. In that order! Sometimes, my mind was spinning a hundred miles an hour. My flight log took a few years off and eventually the girls took over most of my time.

After some time, cars seemed to take center stage. Maybe it was the same with girls. They sort of went hand in hand. Both were the elements of dating!

When you've had a mindset for as long as I did, you do not forget it. It just gets 'cubby holed' and is a little dusty for a while. But it's always there! After high school I had started taking flight lessons. My instructor was Jim Leahy. Jim was the main force behind organizing the Stearman Fly In.

During my very first lesson, I got air sick. It was a new experience for me. However, Jim did a couple aerobatic maneuvers to impress me. I threw up all over the cockpit and myself. I was really rattled. All these years of dreaming and planning… down the drain. I told Jim I guess I was not meant to be a pilot. He did not let me get discouraged. He said that I might get used to flying and get over being sick. So, I kept going and he was right. I never had that problem again.

Once I knew I was over my aversion to flight, my money was becoming a problem. I always paid my own way. I was cash and carry, and things were getting tight.

My parents were pushing for college, so in the fall of 1965, I enrolled at Western Illinois University. My freshman year. Wow! It was filled with drinking, parties, women, and some studies. Pretty much in that order.

My grades were taking a back seat to the women and drinking. I did not really have a clear major and decided to drop out. I was running out of money anyway.

I did not take any money from my parents because when my brother was in college, all I heard from them was bitching about what he was costing them. We were not wealthy. Dad was a house painter. Mom was a homemaker.

I paid for books and tuition from money I had saved working on farms and mowing lawns. I had started working in the fifth grade mowing lawns. Now it is gone, along with my 2 'S' college deferment.

As soon as the Draft Board got the information, I was reassigned 1 'A'. Not long after that, I received a letter from the Draft Board to take a physical for induction into military service. My brother had graduated from college, so now we were in the same boat. He and I took the train to Chicago to see if we were fit and sound specimens for military duty. How about that, we were!

He had gotten married that summer and probably could have gotten another type of deferment. He decided to enlist anyway. He ended up going to Armor Officer Candidate School and was a commissioned officer. A second "lewy." After talking to a recruiter, I decided to enlist rather than take chances with the draft. I took all the tests for pilot training and was accepted into the Warrant Officer Aviation Program. Back then, it was better known as "from high school to flight school." I was in! Signed, sealed, and almost delivered.

I joined the Army Reserve Deferred Enlistment Program. That gave me six months to say my goodbyes AND parrrrrty! Boy, did I party. I wasn't old enough to drink, but had been doing it beginning at age 12 with Dad, Grandpa, and Grandpa's brother, Uncle Willard. Grandpa and Willard always had a pint in their pocket or in the glove box of the car. They would always sneak me a drink. Dad never said anything about this, so I guessed he was okay with it. Mom knew it and it was a very sore subject with her.

One time, back in the '30s, Grandpa, Willard, and their older brother, Clearance, rented motor scooters and were racing over the Fourth Street bridge. Back then, the entire bridge was wood, tar, and gravel. Well, on the downhill side, one of them spilled and took the other two with him. After the wreck, Clearance got up and felt something wet in his back pocket.

He looked at his brothers and said, "I hope that's blood!" It was during the Depression and that pint of whiskey had not been cheap.

Besides sneaking drinks different times, I had also been going into bars and liquor stores since I was fourteen. I had never been asked for an I.D. card until after I was back from Viet Nam and married at age 23. Weird!

Because of this, almost everybody in high school hung around me so I could buy them booze. I told them they could get their own if they would just act like they were supposed to be in the bar in the first place. That's what I did. Don't stammer and stutter, just act like you are 21 or older. Of course, I was pretty good sized and looked mature. Everything helps when you're acting! I must have been a good actor. I was in three high school plays and later, one at Western for a drama class.

Chapter

3

Vietnam was raging and the nightly news was full of it. I suppose Mom got scared about flight school because of Dad being a POW. It did not help that those helicopters and planes were getting shot down like flies.

Mom wanted me to get out of the Flight Program. She enlisted two grandmas, two grandpas, and three great-grandparents to help persuade me. It worked. I talked to the recruiter and changed my enlistment to heavy equipment operator. Mom thought that was good as well as SAFE!

My six months went by quickly and it was time for me to leave for Basic Training. I took the train to Chicago where we were bussed to another train station and placed on a troop train bound for Ft. Campbell, Kentucky. That was home for the next eight weeks. In basic, you learned a "whole lot" in a short period of time. It wasn't all bad and there were some good times too.

Ft. Campbell was home to the 101st Airborne. As we looked out the windows of our indoctrination barracks, all we could see was sergeants 'running' everywhere they went. All the time!

One in particular, was the one all of us said, "I hope we don't get that guy as our DI." Well, guess what? His name was Sergeant Dodds, he was airborne all the way, and he was our Drill Instructor.

All the drill sergeants were pushing for us to go airborne. It was part of their job! We were in formation, waiting to get vaccinations and clothes. We all saw paratroopers jumping in the distance. It was cool, but short lived.

One guy's parashoot did not open. He had what's called a cigarette roll. He plummeted straight to the ground. That was the last straw for most of us. Who would want to go airborne after seeing that?

I never had the inclination for jumping out of an airplane anyway. In the first place, I could fly one. I would rather crash land and take my chances.

Another thing they pushed was OCS. Mainly because most of us had college or a degree and scored higher than normal on all our military testing. So, I bought into this…. hook, line, and sinker. My strong point was math.

I was selected for Engineer OCS at Ft. Belvoir, Virginia. However, my class date was more than two months away. So, I was sent to Ft. Knox, Kentucky and placed at the NCO Academy for Leadership Training. Still waiting for my class date, I was next sent to 11 Delta training (Armored Reconnaissance).

Finally, after that I headed to Ft. Belvoir and OCS. "We come from near, we come from far, we come to get our golden bar." We sang that a lot! What a bunch of crapola!

OCS was fashioned after West Point and lasted six months. I arrived there in February, and it was cold and wet. After the second day, the shit hit the fan. We were treated like crap.

You could only sit on the first four inches of the chair with your back erect at meals, while being bombarded with questions the whole time you're trying to eat. You had to place the silverware at a 45-degree angle across the plate after every bite. You had to chew your food completely (25 to 30 times) and swallow before you could take a drink of water, coffee, or juice. I lost more weight in OCS than I did in basic training.

Whether you were in formation or not, you were constantly having to answer questions. Mostly about military protocol, presidents, leaders, battles, and most anything else. Sometimes you were assigned a specific subject to learn for answers.

Some guys ate this shit up; I did not. One of the Junior Tac Officers came by late at night after drinking and he had his girlfriend with him. I guess he thought this would be fun for her to see. He called a formation outside in the freezing cold and we were all in our underwear. We froze our asses off while he had us recite some stupid shit. We could see her in the car laughing. Very funny!

Another time we came back from maneuvers and were really spent. We had been crawling in muddy and icy water. He made sure we only had cold water for showers. We were given three minutes to get showered and hit the racks. This kind of training was just insane.

The next time he came by late at night, I knew what was coming. He called a formation outside. I slid under my desk and stayed inside while everyone else was out in the cold. Like I said, I am a quick learner.

Another incident I found pretty stupid and cruel was holding our footlockers. It was a lesson to teach us the value of time. We had been caught with the lights on five minutes after "lights out." We were instructed to pick up our footlockers and hold them at arm's length.

After about 30 seconds, you would hear "clunk" as one hit the floor. A few more seconds, "clunk," "clunk," "clunk." At 45 seconds, clunk, clunk, clunk, clunk, clunk. You get the idea. I was with the last three candidates to drop our footlockers. They weighed about 20 to 30 pounds, I guess.

I was pretty proud of that, but of course, we got a lot of razzing about it. Once in basic, Sergeant Dodds dinged me for something and told me to drop and give him ten (do ten push-ups). I had a lot of upper body strength and was really good at push-ups. So, I said, "Is that all, Sergeant?" His face flushed as he hollered, "Gimme 20." Again, I said, "Do you want 50?" He was really pissed! He hollered louder, "Gimme 100, you smart ass." I settled for that and did the 100 with ease. He was right though; I was a smart ass and suffered because of it on more than one occasion.

We had to take a PT test every Saturday in OCS. With a lot of upper body mass, my areas were pushups, sit ups, pull ups, and rope climbing. I was not a good runner. We had to climb up a rope, cross over, and climb down the other side. The candidate next to me was struggling. I swung over to him and helped him make it to the top.

I figured I would get some brownie points for being a team player. Instead, I was criticized and docked on my points. I decided that I would no longer be a team player. Of course, that decision led to some other problems.

I also decided I was not meant to be a 2nd Lieutenant. I was struggling inside with myself. This was that part of mental illness that keeps you awake at night.

I was having a lot of trouble swallowing and would cough some blood every so often. I finally went on sick call one morning. I was admitted to the Army Hospital at Ft. Belvoir and had to have my tonsils taken out. I had some other complications.

After my stay in the hospital, I returned to my company and reported to the CO (Commanding Officer). He stated that I would have to be "set back" to the third or fourth week.

That did not sit well with me. I was not about to go back through all the crap for starting classmen again. I would have been an upperclassman in two weeks. That meant a few privileges and less crap!

I talked with the Senior TAC Officer. We had a long talk. He wanted me to stay, but it fell on deaf ears. I was released from my obligation and OCS.

I was told to report to personnel for re-assignment. Once again, I was on hold. I made the best of it. A 'real' Sergeant E-6 was a candidate in OCS.

We had made a connection our first week. I went back to the barracks to see him. He gave me the keys to his car, said, "Do not wreck it and keep gas and oil in it. When you're finished, put it back where you found it." That was pretty nice of him.

I went to see the sights in D.C. I was still twenty years old and NOT legal, but I went to the bars anyway. I was never carded and drank sensibly so I would not wreck the car. After ten days or so, personnel called me in.

The lady at personnel was a good-looking civilian. She had also been in the Marine Corps. I was on my best behavior, and I think it paid off. She reviewed my records and saw the 11 Delta MOS (Military Occupational Skill).

She stated that's where I would be going. I immediately told her I had not even finished that school. "Please don't put me in that. I didn't pay attention either because I was waiting for a class date for OCS. You'll get me killed if I go into that." She looked at me strangely. She said, "All right, what would you like to do?"

While I was low crawling and miserable in OCS, I happened to notice cars driving by that had to have heaters in them. The two MPs looked warm, and I thought it might be a pretty cushy job. One that would suit me.

I said, "Could I go to Military Police school?" She looked at all my test scores and said, "No problem." She made a couple of phone calls, and told me to go to another office and pick up my orders. I said, "Thank you, ma'am." She said, "My name is Kay." I said, "Thank you, Kay." She just smiled and said, "Take care of yourself."

I picked up my orders and was on my way. My orders read 15 days' leave, two days' travel time, and report to Ft. Gordon, Georgia Military Police School.

I went home on leave and found a couple of old buddies. We went to Peoria for a night out. We did not know it, but the bar we went to was a black bar. Everybody was staring at us, but we were already halfway inside.

Then this older gentleman told the bartender to get us a drink and him one too (on our dime). We ordered beer and he ordered Chivas Regal.

We were standing there drinking, and this old guy reached around my buddy and pinched this gal on the ass. She started raising hell and I figured we were in deep shit. Then, this ole colored guy said, "Hey, these boys with me," and that was the end of that. He was like the head honcho. We finished our drinks and decided to leave.

On the way back to Galesburg, we stopped at every bar on Hwy #150. When we arrived back home, it was time to call it a night. We were loaded.

I left for Ft. Gordon the next day. I got off the plane at the Augusta Airport and caught a cab to Ft. Gordon. I told the driver I needed to go to the MP School. That's where he took me, but to the wrong company. I reported in and the First Sergeant asked why I was late. I said I didn't know that I was. He said class had started three days ago.

He told me to report to the CO. I received an Article #15 for being AWOL, and was restricted to the company area and given extra duty for two weeks. After the following two weeks were up, it was the end of the month and payday.

Except, I never got paid along with everyone else. The CO told me to take his jeep, go to finance, and see what the problem was. I did. I was told that I was not only AWOL, I was listed as a Deserter and dropped from the roles. Therefore, no pay, and I probably would be going to the stockade.

I explained how I had called a taxi at the airport, and he took me to the company. They finally figured out that the taxi driver had taken me to the WRONG company.

I was supposed to report to the company two or three streets over. Had I done that, I would not have been AWOL and none of this would have ever occurred. I didn't think about it at the time, but I probably might not have gone to Nam either. Everything would have been different! You never know!

So, my records were straightened out and I was not in trouble, and I got paid right on the spot. I noticed in later years that the AWOL charge stayed on my record. Just another military SNAFU. Oh well, it wasn't really a big problem.

MP school was eight weeks long and I really liked it. Police work was interesting to me, and I started thinking, hell, I can be a cop when I get out. Not bad! Well, that's a whole different story.

After we graduated, all of us received orders for Viet Nam. We went home on leave for 30 days and met up in St. Louis at Jeff's home. We all went 'out on the town' somewhere in St. Louis.

There were five of us that were pretty good buddies. I mention no last names because they are still alive and it's a privacy matter.

We boarded a flight bound for Ft. Ord, California (our shipping point). We stayed there maybe a week and were on the manifest for the next flight overseas. Now we were headed for Okinawa to get some special training before going on to Viet Nam. It was a long flight. First stop, Hawaii for a six-hour layover.

It was a 14-hour flight to Okinawa. I sat on a hill there looking out to sea. For the first time, it sank in.

Boy, you are a long way from home. It was kinda out there! Ya know? So, we were on temporary duty for the next 30 days. We tried to make the best of it, because Nam was up next.

We went swimming every day and bar hopping every night. We got massages with some extras. We went to steam rooms, Japanese Tea Houses, and snake charmer shows. I don't like snakes. The Habu is a poisonous snake.

At this one bar, the girl was supposed to have a Habu (doubt it). After I went to the can, I noticed the latch on the snake's cage was not hooked. I told the guys and we got the hell out of there, fast. All I needed was a fucking snake crawling up my pant leg. I would have shit myself.

Next, we were on our way to Nam. My spirits were lifted when we boarded a C-123 Air Force Transport plane. What a rickety old bucket, but I loved it. It put me back in touch with my flying agenda. There were no seats except for nets along each side of the plane. When you had to pee, you had to do it into a tube that went to the outside of the plane. Not sure about #2? Dad had mentioned the piss tube, but I never asked about the other.

We all fell asleep at some point. We were awakened by the pilot saying, "If you look out the windows, you will see why we are not landing here." We looked and got our welcome to Viet Nam. All over the ground there were explosions and fires. Everywhere you looked. Holy shit!

We were supposed to land at Long Bin, but had to go to Tan Son Nhut Air Base in Saigon. We landed safely and got off the plane and into a formation. It was 0200 hours and there were buses waiting for us. We were going to be bussed back along Highway #1 to the Long Bin Repo Depo. That's where all the shelling was taking place and Long Bin was under attack. Holy shit! Hoooly Shitttt!

The military in its infinite wisdom was going to drive us by bus into the fray! What is the matter with these people? Damn!

We made it to Long Bin, but suffered some sporadic gunfire and had a few holes in the bus on arrival. No one was wounded! What a relief.

We would stay at Long Bin for a week or two until they decided what units needed us as replacements. It turned out that most of us from AIT went to the 716th MP Battalion (this was an MP Combat Unit). The 716th had three companies: Alfa, Bravo, and Charlie. They also had attached SGs (Security Guards) and detachments of the 527th MP and 52nd Infantry (MP) units.

Three others from our AIT at Gordon and I went to Charlie Co. All the others went to A and B companies downtown Saigon. Charlie company was out by Tan Son Nhut Airbase northeast of the city.

On the second day at Long Bin, I woke up and noticed I had a problem. I was dripping. I went on sick call. I told the doctor and he laughed loudly, "No way, you have only been here two days and it takes up to nine days for gonorrhea to manifest." After he examined me, he added, "Private, you must be a fast worker, it's the clap."

I admitted to him that we were in Okinawa for 30 days prior and I had been with several different women. He laughed again and said OK. He gave me antibiotics and explained how things would go. He also informed me about Army policy. If you come down with 'clap' or another sexually transmitted disease three times, you get an Article #15 and could be Court Martialed. Something to think about, hard!

Much later (after TET), I heard that one of our MPs from downtown came down with some form of syphilis. They could not identify it and sent him to a hospital in Japan. He was told unless they figured things out and it was successfully treated, he would not be leaving Japan. I never did hear the outcome. Pretty sad.

Chapter

4

We lived at Tent City Bravo, next to MACV Headquarters. MACV was Westmoreland and Abrams' baby. The 716th provided security and patrols in the area, especially MACV.

Newbies (us), we were assigned to static posts and did this behind concrete structures called Kiosks. We were there to provide security to structures and personnel living in BEQs, BOQs, hospitals and nurses' quarters. I didn't care for it much. The only good side to it was sometimes we would get duty at a BOQ that had nurses living it. Almost just like stateside duty.

Luck was with me. A nurse and I hit it off, just from saying hello and talking for about twenty minutes. We saw each other for a week or two, then things started going south. A Captain wanted her for himself. He read us the riot act about "mingling with officers" and "vice versa." In order to preserve the 'order', we stopped seeing each other and the rest is history. No one will ever know what could have been.

We also worked the three main gates at MACV Headquarters, five steel guard towers around it plus three Kiosks. Working static duty wasn't for me. I needed to get on a patrol and get out in the open ASAP. The main problem, I was still a newbie.

There was random small arms fire all the time. Snipers, skirmishes, rocket and mortar attacks almost every day and night. There was the constant turbine noise of helicopters plus all the noise from the Airbase. This was all from military fighters, transports, and civilian aircraft coming and going all day and all night. Every day and every night. You get used to it in short notice and just fall asleep.

It's not like the jungle. There, you need to worry when it all gets quiet. At the airbase, it is never quiet. If it went quiet, something very, very wrong was taking place, and you should consider kissing your ass goodbye. It was never quiet.

Our living quarters were pretty nice compared to what guys in field units had to put up with. We had tents with concrete floors. There was one large fan at each end of the 'hooch' along with a refrigerator and table on one side and an open area on the other. That was for our Mama Sans so they could do their work.

These women had 'clearance' to work on base from the Embassy. Each GI paid ten dollars a month for them to wash clothes, shine boots, and keep the hooch clean. We had two maids per hooch and generally sixteen GIs. Do the math. They made about $160 a month ($80 each). Pretty good money for the Republic of Viet Nam.

We had latrines with regular toilets and showers. Like I said, it was probably much better than most. I was grateful that I had not drawn a field unit.

It was not just our area. It was a small community. There were office personnel, clerks, various personnel that worked at MACV HQs, cooks, supply people, armorers, mechanics, a Marine detachment, air force people that worked at Tan Son Nhut, and a Royal Army of Korea detachment.

The ROKs were in formation one day when I was watching. The First Sergeant was dressing down a South Korean soldier. I did not see the soldier do anything that would be considered out of line.

All of a sudden, the 1st Sergeant hauled off and hit this kid very hard right square in the face, knocking him to the ground. The kid jumped right back up, got back into formation and stood at attention. As if, to say, it's alright if you need to hit me again.

The kid was bleeding and never bothered to wipe the blood away. I never saw anything even close to that ever after that in my life. It was insane, I thought. Especially in a combat zone.

One other time, I was talking to one of the Korean soldiers and he kind of encroached into my space. His breath was atrocious. They had a diet of fish heads and rice with fish sauce and kimchi. Jesus, that smell was just too much. I did not want to insult him, so I had to make up a reason to excuse myself. I told some lies, but over the years, I had become pretty good at that.

Military areas are really like little cities. We had a dining hall, a small PX (sundries and dry goods store), a fire station, and a barber shop (more about the barber later). We could also dine at MACV HQ.

They had a fairly large cafeteria set up for the Officers and Generals. MACV was overflowing with high-ranking officers and generals. The cafeteria was truly like a large restaurant back in the states.

So, now you have some insight into what my life was like when I was a young rambunctious kid. My trials as a teen, growing up and entering the 'real world.' Joining the Army and making it halfway around the world.

This period also shed some light on "the tip of the iceberg." Some things to come would be better and many would be worse. From the '50's, "Don't touch that dial!"

After three to four months 'in country', one is no longer considered a newbie. You are now "on board" and your platoon has confidence and trust in you, for the most part that is.

Everyone has pretty much figured out who has your back and who cannot be trusted too much. You get a real good sense of this just observing guys and how they handle themselves in situations that come up.

You knew who was quick tempered and who was laid back. You knew who was a blowhard and who spoke the truth. Nonetheless, we were buddies. We were one!

One time we were having 'guard mount' at the motor pool, getting ready to go on patrol. There was some asshole who was not in our outfit that just kept pushing the limits. He was drunk and really obnoxious.

Clark was a black guy who had been in Nam for a long time, like three or four tours, and he was still there when I left. So, this asshole decided to start fucking with Clark. Clark told him to shut up and get the hell away from our formation. The shithead could not understand English, I guess.

All of a sudden and within the blink of an eye, Clark explodes with a right cross to the shitheads' jaw. His feet flew off the ground, landing him flat on his back and "out for the count." That is the only time I have ever seen anything happen that quick. I think Clark could have been a contender, back stateside. Like I said, Clark had been in Nam a really long time and I do not believe that he planned on leaving until the war was over.

I have never heard one way or the other. No one has ever said anything about him at our Reunions. Maybe he stayed in VietNam. I have checked several records and cannot find anything that says he was killed. So, I just don't have a clue.

I finally made it on patrol. It was pretty routine. I drove around with a Sergeant checking static posts and relieving MPs, if they needed a break. We would also take radio calls that would dispatch us to a bar fight or problem between a VN national and a GI. Sometimes it was just a call about a GI who had stolen something at the Exchange in the Cholon section. We would apprehend the guy and write a DA 19-32 which is a police report. Then we would transport him to the MP Station downtown Saigon and turn him over to them. Just like back home. Sometimes, we would pick up a drunk GI and give him a ride back to his unit. We were nice guys, but most GIs had it in for MPs.

Even though there is a war going on and you are part of it, life goes on. When you have to shoot at the bad guys, it's war time. When the shootin' is over, it's back to regular duty. But then again, it is Nam and nothing is really regular!

When I had not drawn a patrol, my 'regular' duty would be back to static posts or the towers at MACV. A thought that continued to cross my mind in every thunderstorm was about safety and survival.

Here I am in a small solid steel tower about 30 feet above the ground. Isn't this a primary target for a lightning strike? We went through some very bad storms. I never heard of any strikes happening or any GI ever getting killed.

Maybe the towers were grounded somehow? Surely the military was smart enough to consider all these things? Right?

On one of my static posts, I drew BOQ #3. It was a general's villa. It was actually a decent sized compound. Very nice. He also had his own mess sergeant. A very good cook that had been promoted to Sergeant First Class and was considered a Chef. Some people really had it made. Makes me think maybe I should have finished Officer Candidate School.

There was an MP at the front by the driveway of this general's house. He had freedom of movement and a bar stool behind the Kiosk he could sit on.

I was stationed above the kitchen at the back of the house. One time, I noticed someone at the bottom of the stairs. I figured it was the patrol sergeant or the duty officer coming to check on me or as harassment. So, I pretended to be dozing off.

As the shadow approached me, he reached to take my M-16 that was leaning against the wall next to me. I pulled my .45 out of my holster, pointed it in his direction, and asked, "Can I help you, Sir?"

It was the DO. He stammered a little and seemed to (with a shaky voice) say, "No Specialist, just wanted to see if you were okay." I said, "I'm fine, Sir," and he left quickly after that.

An interesting story I heard from an MP in the 720th at Long Bin was a similar one concerning a full Colonel. This MP buddy of mine had a sentry dog. They are trained to attack and kill. They attack soft tissue: your throat, your armpits, and your groin. You will bleed out within 15 seconds to two minutes if they don't rip you to shreds first.

Someone radioed John and told him the Colonel was coming around. John tied his dog up away from his post behind a truck. The Colonel seemed nice enough and visited for a while. Then he asked, "Don't you have a dog?"

John said yes, but he got loose a little while ago. John said that he had never seen a Colonel move that fast, ever. He jumped into his jeep and was gone!

Another time I was above the kitchen at BOQ #3. It was about four or five in the morning, just barely turning daylight. I heard this really weird sound. It was directly overhead. I would estimate 500 to 1,000 feet above the ground. The noise was similar to buzz bombs I had heard on TV World War II movies.

It was a 106-millimeter rocket. The VC would send them in several directions. When the motor runs out of fuel, they fall out of the sky and hit whatever is on the ground.

The top third of this six feet tall rocket is high explosive. After they fall, if they find a target, it is pretty much destroyed. Many would hit open spaces and just put a large crater in the ground. One did just that in Tent City Bravo (where I lived). It left a crater large enough to hide a D – 9 Caterpillar dozer.

I learned later that this particular rocket had fallen on the Missouri BEQ. There were several dead GIs and many more wounded. I shall never forget that eerie sound. Likewise, when it ceased making that sound! That's when it dropped on the Missouri. Not far from where I was on duty. There was a very loud explosion. Unfortunately, one gets the cards dealt! This is war at its ugliest.

Then there was the time that the SFC climbed up the back stairs and asked if I would like a piece of chocolate cake. He had made it that day for his boss. He had it with him and I immediately said yes. It was very good. Maybe the best that I ever had. It was certainly the best I had ever had in the Republic of Viet Nam. Matter of fact, it was the only piece of cake I ever had in Nam. He also took one out to the MP at the front gate.

Then there was the time at BOQ #3, I was at the front gate on Vo Tanh Street. A couple of M-114 Armored Personnel Carriers pulled up. These guys were 11 Deltas / Armored Reconnaissance. If you remember, that's what my assignment was going to be after I resigned from Engineer OCS.

Luckily, I had convinced Kay, that lovely lady at personnel, to give me another school. I felt really fortunate. I could have been one of these guys. They all looked pretty rough.

I don't think they'd seen a shower in a long time. One guy in this group shoved something in front of my face. I think he was looking for shock value. He had a small rope or chain with "ears" on it. They were ears of Viet Cong that supposedly he had killed. That was the inference.

No doubt they were ears from dead people, but who knows if they were killed VC or just some dead person. For that matter, it is possible they were murdered people or VC at the hands of other GIs or worse yet, the ears of non-combatant civilians.

Stranger things have occurred while in the Republic of Viet Nam and every other War Zone. Some guys brought these practices back to the states with them as too much extra baggage! They probably ended up afoul of the law sooner or later. Hard to say.

I met some guys like this in bars and they were nothing but trouble, with a capital T. We would generally end up in a fight. These were the kind of guys that could not escape Viet Nam in its worst form. It is a form of PTSD, but on steroids.

Then there are the plain and simple liars. I was almost drafted. I almost enlisted. I almost got sent to Nam. I had bone spurs. I have an old football injury. Eventually, you get very tired of hearing this shit!

Honestly, I even considered taking off for Canada. Why didn't I? I realized that IF I did that, then some other poor SOB would have to take my place. I could not do that and have someone get killed in my place if it were my time!

So, I did my duty. It's the price of admission into our society and the American Way of Life. We should all be proud to pay it.

Chapter

5

About twenty years ago, I had a license plate on my car that read RVN 6768. You'd be surprised how many people had absolutely no idea of the meaning behind that. To me, it meant something. I was there in 1967 and 1968. It had left some lasting scars. So, it had some real meaning for me. For people to not know, much less care that I was actually in a war and was almost killed, was a little too much and really pissed me off.

When I first returned to the states, I had trouble readjusting. I would get into bar fights over nothing. Then too, I would get into fights over what anyone said concerning something they did not know shit about. When I realized someone was too young, never there, a loudmouth, or a draft dodger, it would lead to a fight.

Most of the time it was with people that did not know shit about Nam. Their stories did not add up or they were repeating stories they had heard from others. You 'know' the shit you hear, sometimes.

I guess I was on a crusade to make people more aware? Hell, even my wife didn't know anything about Nam or what we went through. There is a saying that came out of Viet Nam by an anonymous author. "You have never lived 'til you've almost died, for those who fight for it, life has a flavor the protected will never know." Nothing was ever truer now, in my life!

Now, fifty some years later, almost everything has changed. I'm too old to get into fights. I haven't smoked or drank booze in 20 years or more, yet sometimes, even I have trouble remembering that I was there. That is, until I have a nightmare or hear a loud, unexplained noise, or think that someone is sneaking around my property or up on me, or hear a loud lightning strike. Then, it all comes back, like it was yesterday.

Many nights, I would wake from a bad dream, get my gun, go outside, and walk around my property like I was on duty.

It was hard to shake! As it turns out, writing must be good for the soul. The idea that things come back like it was YESTERDAY, registers loudly. You never forget that kind of trauma, where you were, or when you went through it all. Writing about it helps, in some ways!

From working at one of the main gates at MACV HQs, I got to know a regular visitor. He was a retired Army Lieutenant Colonel working for Air America. Air America was the unofficial Air Corps of the Central Intelligence Agency. I know most Gis are aware of this, but civilians; I doubt it, like I said most of 'em didn't know shit about Nam and what really went on.

I think this guy is dead now. His name was Rock, and, in our conversations, it came up that I had some flight hours and wanted to get into aviation. He invited me to go up flying with him. It was a huge move in my favor.

He even let me take the controls of this Helio Courier Stol aircraft and I had no problems jumping at the chance. My guess is that he was impressed.

He asked what my plans were after the Army. I told him that I would probably go back to college and also, that I really didn't know. He said, "Go home, get all your flight ratings, and file an application with the DAC and CIA."

The DAC is the Department of Army Civilian. They are involved in a lot of things. I would end up with them a little further down the road.

Rock said "the company" would bring me back to Nam as a pilot and start me out at $26,000.00 a year, plus extras. All TAX FREE. This was 1967 and that was very good money. I had every intention of taking him up on the offer, but things didn't work out that way.

I was distracted from my plan. Women! I know Rock had been involved in some sneaky, clandestine stuff that he would not talk about or anything 'the company' was doing. He used to say, "Do you know how to keep a secret?" and then he never said another word.

Back at my MP company, I landed the pipeline patrol. It was out in the boondocks, and we were on our own. Literally, because our radio transmissions were going nowhere out there. So, we could not call for help, if we needed it. No one was going to hear us, and no one was going to show up.

The pipeline ran from the river to the airbase. JP-4, jet fuel, was pumped from barges on the river to a pipeline that ran above ground for about three miles and then went underground the rest of the way to Tan Son Nhut Airbase.

We were the patrol for the three miles above ground. There was a group of ARVN soldiers stationed midway. We would visit them for a while sometimes. One of them spoke English. He had a very badly scarred up head, resulting from hand-to-hand fighting with the VC during an attack somewhere up north. He was lucky to be alive.

Our jeep had a quarter inch of steel armor plating. It was not really bulletproof, but helped ease your mind if you were thinking about getting shot up. My partner was an SG (Security Guard) assigned to our MP unit. He had been in the 25th Infantry and had gotten wounded, then re-assigned with us. When he was being medevaced, he was shot again, in the butt! So, he had two purple hearts. Think of it, he had a 'purple heart' for a bullet in the ass!

We each had an M-16 submachine gun with 10 magazines and both of us carried a .45 caliber pistol with seven magazines.

We had an M-60 machine gun with two boxes of ammunition, 500 rounds each, an M-79 Grenade launcher with 20 rounds, and a case of hand grenades. All in all, we were pretty well armed. We felt safe. Whether we were or not is one helluva big question.

Once, when we were en route to the river to begin our patrol, we strayed off course and visited a house of ill repute. As we left, I got a bad case of the willies and was pretty scared until we figured out what was going on.

All of a sudden, there were soldiers on each side of the road, marching the opposite way we were going. The hair on the back of my neck was standing straight up. I thought, sure, this was IT. Holy Shit!

These guys could attack us at any moment, and they just kept coming. Maybe fifty or sixty of them. They never made any moves in our direction, but we were as ready for something as we could be. As we neared the main road, we saw five or six trucks with several soldiers standing by them.

We figured out this was a "conscription" raid. The soldiers would go to each house, if you were fifteen years old and up, YOU WERE DRAFTED, on the spot. You were loaded in the trucks and taken away to be trained in the Army of the Republic of Viet Nam. Also, the duration of your conscription into the army was until the war was over or you were killed.

After this incident, my gunner mentioned that if we came under attack, we would have to get out of the jeep and set up a defense. I told him, "If you get out of this jeep, you're on your own, I will leave your ass here by yourself. Our radio transmissions go nowhere, so we cannot call for backup and you know it. We would be dead meat!" He thought about that, then said, "Right!"

After TET 1968, I never felt safe again. I was always looking for anyone to make a wrong move in my direction or anywhere around me.

VC and the North VietNam Army were behind every bush, in every building, in trees, and infiltrated into our own units. They had even dug tunnels in a cemetery. We were in deep shit!

We would be able to fight off saboteurs attempting to blow up the pipeline, but not a full-sized assault unit. Remember, we were on our own out there. Mom would have a shit fit, if she knew what I was doing, so I stopped writing after we came under direct attack during TET.

We were on patrol on Plantation Road in the gun jeep. Our QC (Quan San) was riding with us who spoke fluent English. There was also "White Mice," a Vietnamese Police Unit in the lead of our patrol. They turned down this alley in the Cholon Section and our QC said, "Stop, don't follow them; I think it's an ambush." "If we follow them down the alley, we will not come out."

I am absolutely certain to this day that if we had gone down that alley, we would not have survived. Our QC knew the white mice could not be trusted. He was also not Vietnamese. He was caught up in a conscription raid. He said he had explained to the sergeant that he was Chinese. He said that the sergeant simply said, "You Chinese, you live in China. You live in VietNam, you Vietnamese." Logic in its purest form. Who could argue?

Unfortunately, our QC was in the South Vietnamese Army for the duration. He rode with us for a few weeks. After that, I do not know what happened to him. I choose to believe that he had just been re-assigned. There were many people you got to know and would see them for a while and then they would disappear. It is hard to say what may have taken place.

Chapter

6

A week or so after TET, I was on duty at BOQ #1 on Plantation Road. Within a day after TET, Martial Law had been declared for the entire country. The 'curfew' was set at 2200 hours or 2300, I don't remember.

A jeep approached from Tan Son Nhut airbase. It was close to 0100 hours, long after curfew. In the jeep were a full Colonel, a Major, and two Captains. The Colonel was driving. They were all drunk and disorderly. The Colonel hollered, "Hey, Sentry, open this fucking gate." Number one, I was no Sentry. I was a Military Policeman there to provide security for the occupants in that compound. Again, he hollered for me to open the gate. I did not budge or say a word. Someone else hollered, "Open this goddamn gate, soldier." Again, they got nothing from me.

Next, I heard a crash. The Colonel had rammed the jeep into the gate, breaking the lock, and forcing the steel gate open. Once inside, I heard the Colonel state, "I am going to kill that fucking sentry." I firmly believed that would probably happen as they were all armed. I picked up my M-16 and aimed it at the doorway between the compound wall and my kiosk outside. All my weapons always had a round in the chamber, so my .45 was ready to fire also.

As the doorway opened, the Colonel started to move in my direction. I was pointing my M-16 directly at him and was getting ready to shoot. The

Major or a Captain put his hands high in the air shouting, "Hey man, don't shoot, don't shoot, let's all calm down."

I did not know it at the time, but there was a full Colonel either awake or on duty inside the compound and he heard the entire situation. The drunken Colonel who caused the problem had sobered slightly when he saw my M-16 pointing directly at him, it was then he realized that I had never said a word. I was simply poised, ready to shoot him.

By this time, the Colonel from inside the compound, made his presence known, and ordered everyone to "shut the hell up." The reprieve gave me the opportunity to radio my duty officer.

Within twenty to forty minutes, the duty officer shows up. He is a first or second lieutenant. It is only now that I lowered my weapon. I explained to him what had taken place. The duty officer's comment was, "Why didn't you just open the gate?" I stated, "That is not my job, and I was on duty at my post."

The Colonel inside the compound confirmed all that had happened and stated that I had not done anything wrong. It was these four (pointing at them) that are in the wrong.

Of course, the MP duty officer still maintained it would have been much easier to have just opened the gate. *Bull shit!*

After I returned to the company, I was told to report to the First Sergeant. He asked what had gone on out there. I explained in detail. He said to write that all down verbatim and don't leave anything out. He took my statement and said this is an 'official report.' I was glad to hear it. It was the truth.

The First Sergeant said that he was proud of me for standing my ground. He further said, "Most of the guys in this company would have gotten killed or had the shit kicked out of them."

A few weeks passed and the First Sergeant called me in again. He said that he just wanted me to know that if that Colonel "ever" thought he might make General someday, he is sadly mistaken and that those other 'clowns' would probably resign their commissions as soon as possible and disappear from military life. Comforting!

I heard there was a Court Martial. The Colonel pleaded "no contest" and accepted full responsibility.

He was reduced one grade and forced to retire. I never had to appear nor testify. I was too naive to realize it at the time, but booze is nothing more than mental illness in a bottle. It cuts life short, changes ambitions, ruins couples' dreams, and generally wreaks havoc with anyone picking it up. A man takes a drink, the drink takes a drink, and the drunk takes the man.

The only one who actually stood up for me was the First Sergeant. I think the CO, all the officers, and the Provost Marshal must have figured I just should have opened the gate. Normal and the Army marches on!

My brother was a First Lieutenant now. He and his wife were stationed at Ft. Hood, Texas. He was big on Armor and Hood was HIS dream.

Mom had her eyes glued to the news every night after TET. She listened for any sign of my unit. TET was a huge invasion coordinated over the entire country of South Viet Nam. The south is about the size of California.

We had many briefings that intelligence indicated that we could expect isolated attacks during the celebration of TET. This was kind of a standard briefing that we had heard many times. The NVA had a celebration planned for us all right, but it was certainly not a party. It was certainly not what the US had expected either.

All the kids we had been buying Coca Colas from, for the past six months had the real intel. They said, "Buku VC are coming to the south and we will get killed." One kid said to me, "Maybe VC 'kocka dau' you." Kocka dau means, cut your head off. *We knew things were gonna be bad!* The idea of having my head cut off scared the bejesus out of me. I didn't like the thought of getting shot or blown up either.

I guess Mom was calling my brother every day trying to have him find out about me in Viet Nam. She thought he must have connections with the brass. It was all to no avail, he just schmoozed her about how things were going in Nam. Luckily, Mom bought what he was saying. He kept her from worrying too much.

He had no idea and knew he could not find out anything. Things were quiet about what was really happening. That's the way of Washington D.C.! Quiet.

The only ones who knew anything were big shots at the Pentagon, and they were not talking, except for 'the stories' fed to the news outlets. That's how things "really" work.

You all should know this by now. Don't ask a dumb question, you know won't be answered, at least not honestly. And never take anything seriously that is put out by "an official Government spokesman." They lie through their teeth! It's what they get paid to do.

McNamara knew we were in 'serious trouble' after TET 1968. I am told that he went to President Johnson and informed him, "We have to get the hell out of Viet Nam," as quickly and quietly as possible.

McNamara is also the same guy who encouraged the war prior to that, starting with President Kennedy and then with Johnson. I believe Johnson was blindsided by TET and he also realized we were in deep trouble. We should have listened to the French who told us, "Do not get involved in Viet Nam."

The French had lost their entire 2nd Airborne Division of the French Foreign Legion at Dien Bin Phu in the 1950's. They tried to warn us in good faith. Warning Americans just doesn't work.

Congress screwed us GIs in the 1960's. In their infinite wisdom, 'they' had declared Hanoi and Haiphong "diplomatically immune targets;" therefore they could not be bombed. They literally tied the hands of air crews. If Congress had not done this, the war could have very well been over a lot earlier, and we probably could have won the war.

Our gun jeep escorted an M-48 A-1 Tank through the city to a street that was too narrow for it. So, we went in the jeep to this hotel where USAID workers were staying and they were afraid to leave. They had to get out because they were surrounded by hostile forces. The situation could turn bad at any moment. The tank was waiting on the main street for us to return.

We got into a small fire fight with three or six NVA or VC. We killed two of them and the others took off into the night.

We managed to evacuate all 25 USAID personnel, loaded them in a deuce and a half, and got the hell out of there. After we got them safely to the airport, the tank returned to its unit, and we returned to patrol duty.

Supposedly I had been put in for a bronze star, but it had never been awarded before I left Nam. After I returned to the states, I had actually forgotten about it. I had an aversion to medals anyway.

It seemed the higher rank you held, the higher medal you would receive. Especially officers, they would get a bronze star for doing next to nothing, and sometimes nothing at all, literally.

If a SP 4 would get an Army Commendation medal for recognition, while involved in an armed confrontation, a Captain or a Major would get a Bronze Star for the exact same thing.

Maybe even silver. That's the way it worked, and "that" was my aversion to medals. Sometimes, they are nothing more than a very dubious distinction.

I must make this very clear, that most of the time, they are well deserved and well earned by the soldiers they are awarded to. Please do not think that I am being critical of awards and decorations, nor of the men and women receiving this recognition.

I believe that you are intelligent enough to understand my meaning here, at least I truly hope so.

And, in case you don't, there are some assholes who get medals and they do not deserve them. They did not earn them. These are the ones I am referring to!

I have heard it said that Senator Joe McCarthy of Wisconsin awarded himself several medals. Everyone knew he was undeserving of them.

This earned him the nickname of "tail gunner Joe." (It was said that he was sitting so far behind the plane that he could never get hurt.)

This is the same Senator that headed up the inquisition about Communists in government, the movie industry, radio personalities, artists, and more. It was not a shining moment in history.

I was on internal security at Tent City Bravo when the attacks of TET began. It was about 0300 hours on the morning of January 31, 1968. I remember it well, because I was two weeks into being the big 21 and I was not certain I would ever see 22 or the states again. Remember, you get the cards you are dealt.

Our alert truck passed by my post within minutes after the attack began. If you were not on duty, you were on the "ALERT FORCE." It consisted of a lead jeep with driver and Duty Officer. A deuce and a half truck with alert gear (bad idea), driver and duty Sergeant, and 11 to 14 MPs in the back.

That night, I was assigned to BOQ #3, but Jefferson, my bunkmate, wanted to trade. So, I took his post in Tent City and he went to BOQ #3. Jefferson ended up losing an eye during the attack.

Originally, the Alert Force was going to go down Vo Tanh Street enroute to a 'stated' problem at BOQ #3. They had received information that Vo Tanh was lined with explosives, so they changed the route.

At the corner where BOQ #3 was located is a small street, actually an alley, directly across Vo Tanh from this alley was the Joint Armed Forces Chiefs of Staff for the South Vietnamese Army.

The North Vietnamese Army had set up shop in the alley. Other NVA were invading from the far side of this compound. They were supposed to push the military to escape out the front gate. The NVA and the guns in the alley were trained on the ARVN compound, so when all the military people inside came running out to escape, the NVA could kill them all.

Only the alternate route our Alert Force decided to take was a few streets over and then down that alley toward Vo Tanh trying to get to BOQ #3.

When the NVA realized this, they simply turned their guns 180 degrees in order to be head-on with our Alert Force. Now we became their target.

If I remember, the driver and Lieutenant of the lead jeep made it through the alley. They returned to the fight, but could not make much progress getting into the alley. So, they took up positions near BOQ #3.

The NVA sent a B-40 Propelled Grenade into the front right of our two and a half-ton truck, lifting it straight into the air, and then dropping it back to the ground. Then they opened up with machine gun fire and everything else they had.

The casualties on the truck were almost total. Nine MPs from Charlie Company died in that alley during the early hours on the first day of TET

1968. There were other units serving with our company at the alley. In all, there were 21 killed and 28 wounded. Of the 21, 17 were MPs.

The truck had been completely riddled with bullets of all sizes. One of the survivors later stated that the "alert equipment boxes" were in the way and had prevented more guys from getting off the truck. They maybe could have survived also.

I learned three years after TET, that one of the MPs had made it over the side of the truck and had managed to climb up on top of the drive shaft, saving his life. He stayed there from early in the morning until late afternoon. Gunfire was pretty continuous until sometime in the afternoon. Then sporadic. Quite a few reinforcements had been called for assistance.

At some point, I considered praying to God that if He would just let me get out of this alive, I would stop cursing, lying, running with wild women, stop drinking, and become a decent human being. I did not say that prayer.

I did not pray because I think I realized that I would not be able to keep my side of the bargain. Plus, I do not believe one is supposed to bargain with the Lord in the first place. I think He heard that prayer anyway!

I had believed for those three years that Mosley had been killed in the alley. Then one night at Ft. Leonard Wood, Missouri, he stood before me at the MP Desk. It really took me by surprise.

I thought I was seeing a ghost. I asked, "Mosley?" He said, "Yeah, it's me," then we talked, and he explained that he was the one that made it over the side of the truck and onto the running gear. As the firing subsided and our guys moved into the alley, he came out to safety. Amazing, just amazing!

I went to our 50th MP Reunion in 2018. I heard many stories; some troubled me. Guys were saying crap they did not know about. One in particular had given a filmed interview. I heard him mention Mosley and asked what he said. He said Mosley was killed in the alley. I said, no, HE WAS NOT and explained seeing him in 1971 at Leonard Wood. He acted like he did not believe me.

The 720th MP Group sent a V-100 (large, wheeled armored vehicle) from Long Bin to assist us in the alley. It was on the tail gate of this vehicle we had placed our MPs bodies in order to get them out. It was a very sobering experience.

If my memory serves correctly, I think this photo was on the cover of *Time Magazine* in February of 1968. It was this vehicle and the bodies of Charlie Companies' MPs on the back.

When the fighting was over, most if not all the estimated 200 NVA had been killed or taken prisoner. Some escaped into the city.

The NVAs plan to attack fleeing ARVNs from the JAFCS across the street, was not only thwarted by our Alert Force in the wrong place at the wrong time, but by the simple fact that most ARVN troops were not in the compound. They were away celebrating at TET festivals or home on leave.

Hindsight is, most of the time, meaningless. In this case, it had some significance. Vo Tanh was not lined with explosives as reported and BOQ #3 was not really under attack.

If we had known all this, the alert force would not have taken an alternate route into the alley and stumbled into being attacked.

Likewise, they probably would not have been dispatched to BOQ #3 in the first place. But who knows for sure? Not me!

I have one haunting image that has remained in my head since that fatal day of January 31, 1968. While in Tent City Bravo, I noticed a person climbing the water tower inside the Pacific Architects and Engineers Compound at MACV.

I had him in my sights and was ready to fire, but I hesitated. I knew full well the value of the enemy having someone high up on top of that water tower. He would serve to direct mortar and rocket fire. I just could not imagine how the enemy could have gotten into the compound without clearance. Thinking cost you time, and in this case, my target was slipping away.

I likewise could not imagine how or why a GI would be climbing that tower on that particular day. However, just a couple months earlier, I had climbed that very same water tower in order to take pictures of aircraft on the tarmac at Tan Son Nhut. The difference is we were not under attack then.

(About our barber.) He had been issued a clearance to work in our compound. He had given me many shaves with a straight razor. He could have slit my throat and many more when he was our barber. He did not, he was waiting for TET.

He was found lying dead in the rubble of a building destroyed by tank fire outside our back gate. He had been there with the VC or NVA. Beside him lay his mortar tube and several unspent mortar rounds. The intelligence and those doing clearances for foreign nationals, leaves some questions.

I'm sure he had a clearance; I guess I should have shot this guy climbing the tower when I first spotted him. I believe to this day he was probably NVA or VC.

I believe it would have been a fairly easy shot for me. I had always fired 'expert' with several different weapons. It was approximately 250 to 300 yards, and I believed I could 'hit' the individual or, at least, make him fall to his death. I did not take the shot; I should have. It bothers me, but after all this time, would it have made any difference? I believe "No."

First Sergeant Schunck was a World War II and Korean War Veteran. He looked mean with a heavily pockmarked face. He could be mean, but mostly he was strict and a very fair person.

I was in the hooch trying to get some rest. I had been on duty for close to thirty-hours. 'Top' had provided some 'bennies' to help us stay alert and awake.

I had not seen him in a few days, so when he saw me, he said my name and marked a line through it on our roster. That meant I was still alive. He was, at the time, still unsure about this for many in the company.

He asked if I could drive a three-quarter ton. I replied yes and he said, "You have to go to the airfield ammo depot and pick up a load of ammunition."

"They have .50 cals, 7.62 and M-16 rounds, M-79s rounds, .45 cals, and hand grenades for us. Here is an open requisition, get as much as you can get. Tell the ammo supply sergeant it's for me, he knows the situation we're in."

They filled the truck and I headed back. I was by myself. All of a sudden, bullets started zinging off the hood of the truck. One went through the door, but missed me; others went through the canvas top. Theorizing, I told myself, Ho Chi Minh told his guys to shoot us. Our President told us to shoot them.

If this SOB that is shooting at me, would just stop for a minute and pow-wow with me over two or three beers. We could probably work something out, so he wouldn't blow up me and I would not shoot him. Made sense to me.

Of course, the conversation never happened. He did not know I was carrying all that ammo or I would have been blown up by now. End of story. No, I made it back to camp and finally got some rest.

At some point, I was awakened and told to get the jeep and my gunner. We had to go back to where we had rescued the USAID people because an MP from New York was unaccounted for, and he had been with us at the time.

We were just about ready to leave and he showed up. He had gotten sick and had been in the 'head' for quite a while with the shits and throwing up. The story was much more complicated than just that and almost made me sick.

The pipeline patrol had been canceled after TET. It was too dangerous out there alone. We did routine patrols around Tan Son Nhut and the city. A little heavy handed for a gun jeep, but whatever.

Our QC stayed with us. One night, we were on idle time. My gunner had dozed off. The QC, pointing to the gunner told me, 'Do not fall asleep.'

He made his point by saying, "You don't know me, maybe I am a VC spy. If you fall asleep like him, I could easily slit both your throats, steal this jeep, and be a big hero."

I did not fall asleep. Besides, something more was going on in my head, but what? Some demons from the iceberg were moving in and would follow me home.

Chapter

7

I mentioned mental illness as "tip" of the iceberg. Well, more of the iceberg was beginning to show itself. After TET, I was becoming increasingly more paranoid. In addition, I was having bouts of depression followed by manic episodes. In those days it had the label of Manic/Depressive.

I was drinking more and more to alter my mood swings, and I believed for a long time that was working. I was getting so caught up with 'drinking as a cure,' that I failed to recognize just how much harm I was doing to ME.

No one ever noticed and no one even had a clue, because most GIs drink a lot. They also act just like me. My tolerance level was higher than most. I could drink any five guys under the table and still walk straight. However, my brain was suffering, along with my kidneys and most of the rest of my body. It was telling me something I did not understand. So, nothing changed.

The remainder of my tour was filled with skirmishes, rocket and mortar attacks, snipers, and saboteurs. Small kids may have been the worst. If you hesitated to shoot, they were gone and would strike somewhere else. We had enemies everywhere. We had three more 'offensives' after TET. A spring and summer offensive and one more, I don't remember what they called it.

To most people, 'offensives' had little meaning. To me, it meant more than getting a medal. Each offensive represented one battle star. That gave me four. That was three more than most GIs get for doing only one tour of duty.

I finally developed a 'short timer' attitude and I was getting superstitious about going on patrol. I was too far in to get killed now.

I think most guys get this way to whatever degree. Most guys except Clark. I'll say it again. He had been there a long time when I arrived, and he was still there when I went back to the states.

If you are a Sergeant or have re-enlisted, you can figure you might do more than one tour in Nam. I am aware of a handful of GIs who like the thrill and threat there, even if it was dangerous. Some of them had done five or six tours. Go figure.

I would say most GIs, especially draftees, just did one tour. Ironically, even some draftees re-enlisted and became lifers. I guess the Army grew on them.

I did know one guy who was in the California National Guard. Back then, it was a little weird seeing a Reservist and especially, a National Guardsman in Nam. This guy did not go to meetings and finally was activated into the regular army and sent to Nam. He found out the hard way who was in charge.

We had a guy from New York that had re-enlisted for six years in order to get out of the Big Red One. He had written to his mother that he would be safe now. He was given on the job training to become an MP. It is very unfortunate, but he was one of the guys killed in the alley.

A good friend I met in Nam was drafted at the age of 28. We talked quite a bit. He had graduated college, and written and published his first book while in college. It was titled *A Season on A Far Summit* by George Dunbar. Neil Hancock was his real name, Dunbar was a pen name. Neil was successful. He ended up with eight, nine, or ten published books. His style of writing was not for me. He did tell me that sometimes, "You have to disguise your writing," or it does not get published. That's a form of censorship. Get the message?

His personal story is interesting. He was a draft dodger and was married to a hippie. She was also a bitter hippie.

After their divorce, she turned him in to the draft board. It didn't take long and the Board soon caught up with him. At some point, she stated to him that she hoped he would get killed in Viet Nam. Friendly exes are hard to come by. What a nice gal.

Neil was seven years older than me. He seemed like my big brother. He always encouraged me to write. He said, "Everyone has one really good story inside of them and some people have several."

At his age, basic and AIT must have been rough on Neil, but he made it in spite of all odds. He was not in very good shape and was a heavy drinker. That had something to do with why we hit it off so well.

After Nam and the Army, I kind of lost track of many old friends. As for Neil and me, it had been going on twelve years. Wow!

I was with the Federal Aviation Administration and had transferred to Lubbock, Texas in 1979. I was a GS 13 Step 7 air traffic controller. Most of my relatives had been in Unions. I was no different, I was the President of our local. I would end up being fired in the Reagan Purge of August 3, 1981.

I was at an AA meeting at the Central Hub Group. I noticed a guy across the room looking in my direction. He looked very familiar. Then he stood up and started walking over. He was almost here, so I stood up and said, "Georgie Dunbar." He laughed and said no. I said, "I know, it's you... Neil Hancock. Jesus!"

In Nam, Neil had given up regular duty. He became the Company Clerk because he knew how to type and spell. He was First Sergeant Schunck's right hand man and "Top" took a real shine to Neil. They were a team.

I asked Neil how his life had gone. That took more than this first meeting. Before Nam and after, Neil had led a colorful life.

Hancock had lived in the Virgin Islands, New York, Los Angeles, and San Francisco. He had made it and was a published author. Wow! He casually mentioned he had been in prison. Not just any prison.

A Mexican Prison. The kind of prison people talked about. The very bad kind. Holy shit! He said he would probably still be there if it had not been for his grandparents. They had raised him from a young age, due to some problem his mother had.

His grandpa was a banker in Lubbock. He had to pay extortion money to get Neil out of prison and also out of Mexico. Lucky for Neil, his grandparents were well off. I am sure they probably could have bought off someone at the draft board, but Neil decided to pay his dues, even if it meant Nam and the possibility of getting killed.

Neil wrote at night, sometimes all night, and slept late into the day. He said he was awakened by banging on his door one morning. He answered the door and two guys flipped out badges. They stated they were with the FBI and needed to talk to him about all his requests to the Pentagon concerning the records in Viet Nam.

He explained that he was working on a book about the 716th MP Battalion during the TET Offensive of 1968 and that was part of his research. After a somewhat long talk, he said he guessed they were satisfied and left. However, they left open the possibility of further questions in the future. Pretty much just like in the Army!

We had many visits in Lubbock and then Neil moved to another home he had in Houston. We kept in touch after that, first by phone, then by letters, and finally by email.

We were both into motorcycles and did a lot of riding. Neil rode a BMW, and I was into Harleys. We both loved old cars. His were Cadillacs and mine were Corvettes.

His grandpa had given him a 1968 Fleetwood. Neil had taken it to a shop in New Mexico to have it restored. The guy ended up stiffing Neil on the money end and never did any work on the Caddy.

Neil said he had some biker friends who could probably get the money and the car back. The way Neil sounded, I'm sure these guys were part of an outlaw biker club. Neil said their methods were a little crude. Ha!

Neil eventually got married again. He said it was a good marriage. This wife had also been a hippie and a big protester during Viet Nam. Ironically, her father had been a medical doctor in WWII. He had been assigned to Nagasaki, Japan after the war to study the effects of the Atomic Bomb on humans. Gruesome!

Neil died in 2013. He was on his bike and had an aortic aneurysm while he was riding in New Mexico. His wife told me they said he was dead before he hit the ground. I felt bad, even though Neil had had a good life. I miss him.

Neil sent me a picture once of a stork trying to swallow a frog. The frog was in its mouth while choking the stork by the throat. The caption read, "DON'T EVER GIVE UP!" I loved it.

My depression and manic episodes were surfacing again. I saw a shrink. Their big opening question is (always), "Do you want to harm yourself? Do you want to harm others?" My answer was generally, "Do you think I would tell you if I did?"

I had to go to the emergency room in Iowa City. The nurse was a cute gal and she asked me the same questions. I looked at her and smiled. Concerning the second question, I said, "I've got a whole goddamn list at home." I winked at her and she just laughed. It was not reported. At least she had a sense of humor!

So, my iceberg was gaining strength, but I was determined to never start boozing again. I did stay on the meds the VA was providing. They seemed to work.

How I managed to quit drinking in the first place was a wonder in itself. I quit once for two whole weeks and relapsed. Next, I managed to stay off it for six months and relapsed.

Next, I went to a recovery ward in a hospital. I was there for 40 days and it was double full of AA meetings. I hated them, but we all had to attend as a group. When I finished treatment, I was advised, "Do not hang around with old friends," and "Do not go to bars. Go to a meeting every hour, if you need to." I guess the counselor never caught on how much I hated meetings. I hated saying, "Hi, I'm Mike and I'm an alcoholic." Worst of all, I hated hearing it said 20 more times at a meeting.

Hidden within all my problems was a huge problem with my family. I was losing them and did not know it. They suffered much more than I was aware, and it was no fault of theirs. Nam had some effect concerning my singularity and being with many women. That followed me home also.

I did a lot of research and read many books about alcohol and psychology. From alcohol poisoning to studies conducted in Sweden with orphans placed with alcoholic and non-alcoholic families. Both groups fared about the same. I read about abusive drinkers and loss of control drinkers. What was I?

I ended up doing everything they said "do not do" while in the hospital. I went to bars and I hung out with old friends. The big difference was, *I did not drink*, but no one caught on for quite some time that I was not drinking.

I drank plain tonic water with a twist of lime. My secret weapon. It was all part of my plan. I did not need AA and I grew to like the tonic water and lime.

While sitting in bars, as the night dragged on, there I was with my fifth or sixth tonic water. I watched the same people get into the exact same argument they were in the night before.

I watched others get into fights over the same thing they fought over the night before. It was amazingly bizarre.

I watched as they tried to hustle the ladies, with old pickup lines. The ones that didn't work. All you needed to ask was, "Do you wanna get laid?" That worked!

Before my very eyes, I witnessed the absolute stupidity of mankind blossom. Then it hit me, I was those very same stupid individuals, only tonight I was not drinking and NOT GETTING STUPID! This is about the time it registered that "but for the grace of God, there go I". So, this is it! AA did play a part in it after all.

Most of those bar flies would have trouble remembering what took place the previous night. A sober man without medical memory loss has no problem. After approximately four years of doing my brand of treatment, I had become that sober man. I did not want to drink and it did not bother me that others do.

I also learned that I never should have been drinking in the first place and I was actually not an alcoholic. I was bipolar and the drinking years had just made all the problems that much worse. Maybe the iceberg was beginning to melt. To a degree? A little?

Now I had new problems. I was out on a limb as a fired air traffic controller. As I later discovered, I had also been black listed. So, I called some old friends who told me to contact the DAC. Remember them?

I had to leave my family in Texas, because this was an unaccompanied tour. I packed my bags and went to Nigeria, Africa. My choices were Amman Jordan, Costa Rica, Central America, or Africa.

I flew a C 337 Skymaster with a camera. We quietly flew around the country taking pictures for DMA. They are a group in St. Louis known as the Defense Mapping Agency. Maybe a little hush, hush.

The pay was very good. I was paid in Naira and my wife received a check every month from Virginia. It was similar to the army, and I earned three days a month of vacation. If I became ill, I would be sent to a hospital in Germany or Sweden for treatment.

We lived in a German compound in Ikeja, where most of the hospitals were open air and did not appear to be too sanitary. I am sure there are much better hospitals downtown in Lagos. Anything and everything you might want could be found in Lagos. It was a lot like Nam.

It is a peculiar thing, but I do not remember seeing any lightning bugs on Okinawa or in Viet Nam. Maybe I was just too busy with the war to notice. Then, maybe they were staying underground until the war was over.

Now, I am sitting outside our flat in Ikeja and I just realized that I have not seen one lightning bug in Africa either. This is weird. I checked an encyclopedia and there are various species of lightning bugs on every continent. So, where are they?

We had gotten into a little trouble after airport security discovered guns in our plane. We were put in a local prison for two weeks. After this news made it back to the company, it was arranged for bail (or a bribe) to be paid. What a relief.

I now had a very good idea how Hancock felt in that Mexican prison. Our bail was not without a cost. We were summoned to the Embassy.

Pickering was the Ambassador at the time. His staff suggested that we find a way out of the country as soon as possible. We had a little help planning the trip!

Our departure was arranged. We had no exit visa and therefore could never return to Nigeria. What a relief! I wasn't planning on going back anyway.

We really did not receive a warm welcome back in the states either. We were debriefed in Virginia, fired, and sent home. We lost everything we could not carry by hand. Everything we had taken to Africa when we were deployed.

For me, it was a small part of my life. A portable typewriter, two manuscripts I was working on, canned goods, clothes, and souvenirs. Along with some money I had managed to cubby hole. Quite a bit of money. A lot of money.

Chapter

8

When I was home with my family in Texas, my paranoid side followed me. I believed I was being targeted. I was not afraid for me, but for my family. I stayed up all night and slept during the day after my wife had gone to work and the kids were at school and the babysitter.

I was watching a news feed. It was not your primetime variety. You can pick up some real news in the wee hours of the morning. They were interviewing the President of Bolivia. The newsman said, "El Presidente, you know who the drug dealers are and where they are. Why don't you have your Army go and get them so that the drugs do not make it to the United States and into the hands of our children?"

The Presidente was pretty sharp. He knew he was being played. His response was, "Yes, that is true, I know all this, but your President also knows who the drug dealers are in America and he has a much bigger Army than I have. Why doesn't he tell his army to go get them and protect your children?"

The newsman knew that he'd been HAD. He never said another word about drugs and moved on to the country's labor force and the economy.

Another early morning story was about a guy holed up in a motel room in Montana. In the interview, he said that he had worked for the CIA, and he believed that they were trying to kill him. Three days later, the same news person said that guy had been found dead in his motel room.

The news agency contacted the CIA, and an official government spokesman did the talking. He stated that they had NO IDEA who this person was.

He had never worked for the CIA, but they did know that he had a terrible alcohol and drug addiction problem. What a coincidence?

I had a funny feeling and started moving around the house about three that morning. The hair was up on the back of my neck and I felt like something was up. I saw a guy out in front of my house. I could see that he had a full beard and was wearing dark clothes with a baseball cap. Suspicious!

My Viet Nam perimeter guard status took over. I put on a pair of long pants, shoes, and shirt, and went outside. I also stuffed a .357 magnum in my belt. It was very surreal. I expected trouble. I kept my hand on my gun the whole time.

I walked across the street to confront this individual. As I got closer and about to say something, he said, "Hey! I didn't know you were back!" It finally hit me who he was. We talked for a little while as he kept watering his lawn. Likewise, I did not know he had grown a beard. I could have easily shot him.

It turns out this guy was my neighbor. To this day, I have never figured out why in the hell he would be out watering his lawn at three o'clock in the morning. Strange! But then, he was a little strange.

It also seems pretty strange that if the guy in Montana had never worked for the CIA, and they did not know who he was. Then how were they so aware that he had an alcohol and drug addiction problem? Strange?

It is said that truth is stranger than fiction. Many times, people have asked me about what I did for a living. They are looking for some excitement in their lives. Most of the time, I would actually tell them the truth. They would laugh, say, "Yeah, right," and "Let it go." Just goes to show ya!

My cousin Bob had a good saying. When he thought someone was snooping, he would say, "That's confidential…." He would pause, and then say, "That's a nice way of telling you, it's none of your fucking business!"

I always had trouble with too many people asking too many questions. They had no reason to know. Many of them were not smart enough to know when to shut up or to realize you were not talking. Can't they take a hint?

After a few months, I calmed down enough to go looking for a job. I was not satisfied with most of the ones offered, so I started a painting service.

I did fairly well, and it led to some other repair work. Eventually, it led to re-modeling houses for a rental holding company.

Truth of the matter was, I was growing tired of Texas. So, in 1985, I went back to Illinois and looked for work. Whether or not I found work, I had it in my mind that I needed to move home.

We had lost a son in Texas and that was a sore spot. He was buried in Illinois, so the move made a lot of sense to me.

In 1986, we moved to Naperville. The city was growing by leaps and bounds. So was the housing industry. I was part owner in a classic car company that restored mostly Corvettes. I was also in the real estate business. Things were going very well.

Chapter

9

The irony of this massive display by Reagan, against the air traffic controllers, was that he stated many, many times on the national news that Lek Walesa of Poland was a HERO. A 'hero' for organizing the strikes at the shipyards in Gdansk.

Walesa was a hero and American Air Traffic Controllers were criminals. We did the same thing as Walesa. We went on strike. The U.S. is very hypocritical that way.

Another slap in the face was the fact that Reagan rode on the back of unions to get into the Governor's Office of California. He was a Democrat at the time. After he was 'IN,' he switched parties. What a putz!

I do not know if this is true, but I did hear it from a Postal Worker. The word was that postal workers and letter carriers were talking strike. It would come on the heels of the air traffic strike.

In order to scare the postal actions, the government decided to slaughter the air traffic controllers. They would sacrifice 18,000 ATC workers in order to forestall a strike with 700,000 postal workers. DO THE MATH! Apparently, it worked, postal workers never went on strike. Were they afraid, or was some kind of deal made behind closed doors? I just don't know.

What I did know for certain in 1993 was that I was completely out of options and my days as an Air Traffic Controller were over. I further knew that I had been 'blacklisted.' I was running short on proof, and I could not afford an attorney to go against the government. You know as well as I do, Uncle Sam held all the cards!

In 1993, President Clinton lifted the ban against "fired air traffic controllers." Many were re-hired and managed to save their pensions. I was not one of them. I loved that job, and I wanted it back. It was about my entire life's work.

I arranged to retake the battery of tests for ATC. This was easily done due to the fact that I was a disabled veteran. I "aced" the test, scoring over 100. I figured I would be hired within a couple of months.

I was not, so I wrote to the Great Lakes Regional Office in Des Plaines. I received a letter stating that "It has been determined that you are not a suitable candidate for Government employment." What the hell does that mean? Now, I was hot and did some hard thinking. How would I get to the bottom of this! I had to find out somehow.

When I was in Texas during 1980, the Southwest Regional Vice President of the Professional Air Traffic Controllers Organization and I went to the Southwest Regional Office to review my records.

We ran across one page that stated that a guy named Kemp from ACE 610 (an investigative arm of the government) was sent to Davenport, Iowa. He was sent to Mercy Hospital where I had gone to an alcohol treatment facility back in 1977. Kemp was directed to 'attempt' to obtain my medical records (by any means) and return to the RO in Des Plaines.

What the hell was going on? We asked for a copy of my records. The lady left the room for approximately four minutes. She returned and said, under her breath, "I have been instructed to inform you that *your records cannot be located.*"

Well now, what do you know about that? They completely disappeared in four minutes. We left empty handed. I was trying to figure out why are "they" fucking me over? Something was up; I just could not figure out what.

Later on, in 1993, it sort of started to come together. I had been instrumental in planning before the 1981 strike. Could this have something to do with it?

After being fired in August of 1981, a U.S. Marshal came to the Central Labor Council building in Lubbock, Texas. He gave his speech and then said he would be back in a week with a warrant for the arrest of myself and the vice president of our local. He made a nasty comment on the way out. He turned, looking directly at me and said, "Your ass is going to Big Springs Penitentiary."

Sounded personal to me, but this could not be the 'what.' It was probably just due to his being overworked or maybe 'pissed off' at controllers in general.

A week later, he failed to return and no arrest warrant was ever issued. A Federal Judge in Arizona said he was not satisfied that what Reagan was doing was legit. He refused to issue any and all warrants against air traffic controllers.

Other judges across the country followed suit. The arrests were over, but Reagan's "purge" would remain permanent. We discovered this after the one-year mark. All appeals were failing and legal was going nowhere.

Early on in the strike, headlines were made in West Virginia. Federal Agents were shown dragging Steve Wallert out of court handcuffed and in chains. There were four to six controllers that had been tried, convicted, and sentenced. They were serving one year and a day in Federal Penitentiaries across the country. We had become a "target" for America.

That made it all right for Americans to hate us. Pilot Unions and unions in general refused to honor the strike. They treaded frivolously across our picket lines. What assholes!

Thankfully, stewardesses of some unions got together and had a one-page ad published in the Wall Street Journal, supporting "controllers." We were really limited in support, and welcomed theirs because they were part of our industry. They were the greatest!

What President Reagan did to "bust" the strike was illegal and worse than what we did by striking against the government. Reagan used active-duty military to work in towers as strikebreakers. Using the military in civil disputes is illegal!

Maybe he got the idea from President Woodrow Wilson and John D. Rockefeller Jr. in the Ludlow Massacre. The coal miners in Ludlow Colorado were striking. Wilson called in Federal Troops to bust the strike. They shot strikers and set their living quarters on fire. Several were killed, including women and children.

Having unqualified military personnel working the towers and at radar facilities undoubtedly was responsible for causing crashes and loss of life. But who was keeping track? The FAA and Department of Transportation were supposed to be. Instead, they reported everything was running safely. Afterall, they were in collusion with Reagan's decision about letting the military stand in for striking controllers.

It also occurred to me that if we were still under British rule, we would not be in this predicament. Individuals in government employment in Britain who are in Unions have the same rights as regular citizens. They have the right to strike.

After the Marshal did not return, my ass would not be going to Big Springs Penitentiary, as he had stated. However, I was still "blacklisted." This was a very sore spot with me.

I would spend countless hours over my remaining years trying to figure out why they (the Government) would do anything and everything to destroy my career along with my dream and life's ambition in aviation.

My friends, the lightning bugs, would remain the constant source of my inspiration. I watched them every night during the summer.

They would also console me in these rough times, as it seems, no one else gave a rat's ass about my life and its meaning. Reminds me of coming home from Viet Nam.

I came back to the states, but I never really came back home from Nam! I am aware that I am not alone in this nightmare of not coming HOME.

I am 76 now and have given up on finding out about the blacklist. It most likely resulted in the FAA finally obtaining custody of my medical records from the alcohol treatment facility in Iowa.

It would make sense that there was something there that had to do with my state of mind and overall mental condition. Yeah, that was probably it! Case closed. Or is it? Time is no longer on my side. And Uncle Sam NEVER says 'uncle.'

Chapter

10

Sometimes when you think things are coming to an end, it switches and becomes a new beginning. Letha had a second child in 2001. She kept her.

In a song by Glen Yarbough, are the lyrics, "Each time a baby's born, the Lord says 'take it one more round.'" I hung onto that. That little girl was the love of our lives.

Our oldest daughter, Letha developed symptoms of mental illness in Texas at an age between six and ten. I fought it because I *did not* want that to be the case. I refused to believe it and decided to believe that she would grow out of it. The years to come would be very painful.

She did not grow out of it. Her problems grew worse. I did not understand mental illness. I knew nothing about it. I only knew that I had my own problems.

I had been in Africa and had my own disaster. I struggled when I returned home. I decided to move back to Galesburg and then to Naperville.

We tried to get help for Letha from everywhere we could think of. She was finally placed at a mental hospital in Peoria. This was supposed to be a secure facility.

She escaped from there and was gone for three or four months. It seemed like a year. She was in a bad state of health when the police located her. Her problems continued to grow in Naperville.

She was then placed in a hospital downtown in Chicago and she was pregnant. After she came home, it seemed like things were going better. Once she started feeling better, she decided she did not need to take her medication any longer. That was a disaster, but is often the case.

We had convinced her to give the baby up for adoption. We knew that she could not take care of a child. We could not because we were both working. Adoption seemed the only solution at the time.

People who stop taking meds make things much worse by getting into a revolving door situation. They are on meds and then quit. Back on and then quit. She was caught in that door.

Letha's problems had grown full blown now and she had run away for a second time. We only knew she was somewhere in Joliet. She was in trouble and the people she was with were attempting to prostitute her.

She broke away and called my mom from a grocery store. Mom paid for a train ticket to Galesburg. It was waiting at the Joliet Train Station.

Letha asked Mom to help her, but not to my liking. Mom assisted her with getting supplemental social security income for having a mental disability.

That really pissed me off for years because I failed to recognize that she actually was mentally ill and had symptoms of many disorders. We had failed to get her the help she needed. It is a very desperate situation, and you feel totally helpless.

It also presents a black eye for the system. Sometimes it feels as though they do not care or maybe just do not care enough. Things also slip by them because mentally ill people are not stupid, and many times, they outsmart the care providers. However, I do not believe that parents expect too much in the way of care and treatment for these individuals. They truly need help, but the system often fails them.

I thought for many years that our daughter was just lazy. I hounded her about getting a job and making friends to no avail. That had to be the answer to getting her out of this living hell.

At least, it seemed to work for me. I always held a job and seemed to have friends. Maybe this was all just in my head, but it was the glue that was holding me together over the years.

It was not to be for Letha. Her problems continued to manifest in many different ways. She was having a horrible time, struggling with life. She had no life!

My wife turned to religion, finding some peace about it, and managed to accept it. I did not until it began to sink in around 2003. After all those terrible years, I admitted to myself that I had been wrong. Although I still struggled with the idea, I knew that I had to accept that our daughter really was mentally ill.

I finally recognized her symptoms and 'had' to accept what I was seeing. It bothers me a great deal that we could not get help for her.

She is 52 now and leads her own brand of life. It works for her, so who am I to question or advise? Besides, I still fight my own demons now and then. Often!

Our second daughter was born in 1979. Thelma was a fireball. Well mannered. Always doing wild and crazy things. Her ambition was to be a 'Solid Gold' dancer on the TV show by the same name. She was actually pretty good. She became proficient with the violin at an early age and then quit after a few years. The teacher said, "Do not push it," so we let it go. She did not return. Thelma always had good grades until her freshman year in high school.

Something was changing. She was having a lot of difficulty. I did not know it at the time, but she was being bullied at school by a girl gang. The school counselor never mentioned anything about this either. He did, however, advise her that she could 'quit' school at 16 years of age without her parents' consent. Very nice and professional of him. Right?

So, that's what she did. Staying at home alone was not productive in any way. Boredom soon became a problem. Next some mental instability surfaced. Finally, there was an attempted suicide.

She was placed in a mental facility. I believe she was there for a month to six weeks. After she was released, the very next morning, she was gone! She had taken off with two kids she met at the hospital.

This really caused problems for my wife and me. We believed the worst was about to happen again and we could do nothing about it.

Thelma and her friends were located within 24 hours three states west. Had they not been, all parents involved, at least us, believed they would end up dead. Children who do this have NO IDEA just how lucky they are to survive that situation.

Thelma was very problematic for two or three years. Then as quickly as things changed, they changed for the better.

She took her GED and succeeded in getting into college. She graduated and became a registered nurse. We were extremely proud. It seemed she had overcome whatever was standing in the way previously. I believe Thelma has a handle on everything today.

I mentioned we had a granddaughter born in 2001 to Letha. She was a very well-behaved baby. Seldom cried and slept well. Rachel was with us often in Naperville. Most of her life actually.

In '99, I lived between Naperville and Oneida. I bought ten acres from Mom, built a large barn, and finished half of it for temporary living. In 2004, my wife moved and we lived in the barn while they built the house.

As I said, Rachel was with us almost all the time. We ended up adopting her in 2006. We convinced Letha this would be best. She was simply overwhelmed with responsibility. Her intentions were good, but her ability was not.

It was a couple years later, and my wife mentioned that she had noticed some disturbing things Rachel was doing. This continued to get worse. We had gone through 28 or more years with Letha's problems. Now, it seemed it was all starting over again.

Rachel was considered an "at risk" child and began school a year early. She did well at first and our hopes were high. Then things grew worse, at home and at school. She was having difficulty with students and teachers. Rachel could not control her behavior.

We began counseling. The psychiatrist placed her on meds. That did not go over well, and we would find them under the mattress of her bed. She had so many reasons why she would not take them, just like her mom before her. This is a very common scenario when dealing with mental illness.

Rachel was threatening to do some very bad things at school and carried out many threats at home. She was in and out of mental wards at hospitals six to ten different times. This was between ages six to eight.

Next, she received her first suspension at school. At age seven, I took her to a hospital in Chicago. The system is unwilling to place labels on children's problems. Because of this, they do not have a diagnosis.

Rachel was given every test for everything we read about, or was suggested to us as well as any ordered by counselors. All of this wears on a child.

One test, for Augsberger Syndrome, was said to be inconclusive. This test cost two thousand five hundred dollars and we were provided approximately ten pages that literally said nothing. What the hell did we pay for, the paper and copier?

We took her to Springfield for special testing of brain function. When Rachel was living with her mother at age two to three, she had fallen out of bed onto a hard wooden floor two different times that I am aware of.

We thought maybe she had some brain trauma. I believe the conclusion of those tests did not definitively show anything either. Makes you wonder why the hospital agrees to all the testing. For money?

We were striking out again. Rachel had a propensity for matches and fires. She set two fires in our house. They did not become serious. Lucky!

She kicked holes in walls and once slammed her bedroom door with such force, it came partially through the threshold. I had one helluva time getting it open.

She also liked knives. This is a pattern she shared with her mother. However, with a knife in hand, Rachel threatened to kill me if I ever went into "her room" again. That incident got her three weeks on a ward for mental evaluation. Nothing ever comes of these evaluations. I do not know why they waste our time with them.

We never actually received any meaningful information from hospitals, counselors, her psychiatrist, her psychologist or test results. We were coming to the end of our rope again.

We got her into a Baptist Children's Home down state. We visited once a month for a couple hours. The trip was an eight-hour drive. It started out that they would keep her through high school. At eleven months, they called me and said she had to go, she was kicked out. They had sworn when she was admitted that they could help her. She came back home and never received the help they promised.

We talked with a local minister who was also the principal of the church school. They accepted Rachel and we had a little more hope. She was uncooperative and disruptive.

I don't believe it was even four months and we were told she had to go. Things were getting very desperate. I think things were worse with Rachel than they were with her mother.

With nowhere else to go, we got her back into the local school system. The one that had expelled her. She was just there, not really making any progress or doing her homework. That school system would not provide for special education because that cost them too much money. So Rachel was left to stagnate. So much for states really trying to help with the mental illness crisis. It is all just "lip service" and bull shit.

Rachel began disappearing for hours at night. She was eleven or twelve now. Then she began running away. The police were called and they would ultimately locate her. Sometimes they would bring her home. Mostly, they would call us at all hours to come and pick her up at the station eight miles away.

Rachel was very physical with my wife, and in 2013, it came to a head. I was also a big part of a problem that had been brewing for several years. I had not been a good husband. Rachel and I both had mental problems, but that is no excuse.

My wife moved out. She had simply turned the situation "over to God" and freed herself of it. I cannot begin to understand this logic. Rachel continued running away. She was not running from anything in particular. She was just running.

With my ex gone, I was left to care for Rachel on my own. It hit me that sooner or later she will be successful with running away. She would get a ride and be gone. But with whom, a murderer, someone who would prostitute her or use her as a sex slave.

They are all real and they are all out there. Everywhere around us. Most people choose to ignore the facts while others are very naive and just refuse to believe this.

I had no influence and I had totally lost control. Worse, I could no longer provide for Rachel's safety. I was being forced to do something that I really did not want to do. My ex was there during this last run away.

Rachel sat in the back of the squad car with the window cracked so she could talk to us. She, again, had no idea as to why, but she kept saying that she wanted to go to foster care. She believed that magically life would be different.

She told the police that every time they brought her back here, she was going to run away again. It struck me that she was telling the absolute truth. I asked the officer what was I supposed to do, handcuff her to her bed? He smiled and said, "I can't tell you to do that!" Not much help.

The worst had just happened. I told the officer, "That's it, she is locked out." Meaning that Rachel could no longer stay here. I told Rachel, "I do not think you are going to like what is about to happen to you." She had no way to comprehend what I was talking about.

The Department of Children and Family Services was called. Now it became their responsibility to do something with her. They talked with me until five in the morning, trying to get me to allow her to come back home. I did not. That is what we had done so many times before and it never worked.

I knew that we would get into trouble, but I also knew that Rachel would become a "ward of the state" and therefore get the help she needed. At least, that's what I thought would take place. I stood firm. She was locked out.

DCFS does not provide you with too much information because I think that they really do not want you to know what all services are available. Available to them as a state agency.

If you manage to find out somehow, you will be shocked. It costs a parent up to $60,000.00 a year to house an individual at a school facility providing counseling and care. That's out of your pocket.

I was aware of this because I overheard a counselor talking about it. The comment was made that "we, meaning DCFS" can get them into a school, facility, group home, or whatever we need without much trouble, just because we are a state agency.

I remembered this the last time Rachel ran away and my decision was made. It was the only way I knew to get help for her. Rachel was in foster care very briefly. It did not go well. She was at risk of something terrible happening.

Rachel was doing and saying some very disturbing things while in foster care. It ended when the foster parents wanted her out of their house. Rachel's case worker spoke with me and asked if she might actually carry through with some of these things. My answer was, "Yes, I believe so."

The decision was made to send her to a locked facility in Champaign, Illinois. Early on, she did escape somehow, but being a state agency, the cops react much more quickly than when getting a call from a parent. She was caught within twenty minutes. I think that ended her ideas about running away.

She was there for two years. We could visit once a month for two hours. We had some hope again. It seemed she was making progress. On our third or fourth visit, she hugged both of us and said we had no idea how much she loved us. It seemed she was actually at peace with being there and had gained some respect for us. That really felt good!

I'm sure it was genuine. Our visits went more smoothly after that, even though there was always a state worker present. That was okay.

The second year, Rachel had to have an operation. During this procedure, I was given extra time with her and stayed all day. She was my scared little girl again.

After two years, she was moved to a group home in Centralia. Visitation remained the same. This was a four-and-a-half-hour drive. There was no choice, we had to make the trip. Rachel's wellbeing was at stake.

It seemed that my ex-wife was not really comfortable around Rachel; maybe she sensed something. At some point, my ex decided not to visit her any longer. I never knew what that was about. I continued the visits by myself, and everything seemed alright to me.

Rachel was about to turn 18. She had graduated high school five months early. I was proud of her. She was still under control of DCFS, which I never fully understood because they stated that she could leave with whoever she wished and go wherever she wanted after her birthday.

That is except for me. They continued to infer that if I came to take her home, I would be arrested and placed in jail. I took their word for this and tried to work with them.

I bought a house that they approved. They finally stated that she could be released to my custody and the placement would be considered an approved placement by DCFS. To this day, something about this smells fishy and illegal. However, I did not need any trouble in my life.

I truly believe that Rachel had become what is termed "institutionalized" over the last four years. This is exactly why I did not want to have to do this in the first place and I felt very guilty. When she came home, she began living in just her room and did not leave the house, ever. Not even for a walk.

It was extremely noticeable that her life was in that one room. She did not socialize and finally stopped talking with me.

We were at a loggerhead. We were getting into physical altercations. I had to call the police. The second time, Rachel was removed and taken to live with her birth mother. That did not last very long either. Letha also said that Rachel stayed in her small room continuously. Not really antisocial, but not social either.

I do not believe that she is ever going to pull out of this. I think that she will end up like her mother.

We failed all of our children in getting the help they needed in a timely manner in order to provide them what was needed. The system failed them in a much worse way. It is a state agency with a mandate to provide the care, treatment, counseling, and psychiatric care necessary to help these people become productive citizens.

Failing that, they should be required to assist in providing a modicum of care to fulfilling the goal of life, liberty, and the pursuit of happiness.

Most of us treat these individuals as lepers. It's hands off and don't get near them. They are human beings and God's creatures, just like everyone else on this planet. Judge not, lest you be judged! People seem to forget all that in short order.

When some political candidate declares that HE/SHE is going to increase funding for mental health. Do this and do that. In the end, it is all just campaign rhetoric and falls short of any substantial endeavor.

You know it and I know it, so we all should simply call a spade a spade and forget trying to glamorize it for the press. Mental health has NEVER been addressed properly and I feel confident it NEVER will be. It is totally misunderstood. A truthful psychologist or psychiatrist will tell you that we really do not know diddly about it. It is all a mystery.

I can never understand why God took my infant son nor why He allows some children to have severe disabilities, deformities, mental illnesses, and terminal illnesses. It seems cruel that this happens.

Some preachers say we should "praise" God. Some say we should "fear" Him. All of them say we should "pay homage" to Him. They mean "pay money." Makes one wonder why God does not strike some of them dead, right in front of everybody.

Preachers, for the most part, are very hypocritical and never give you a straight answer. They also like to increase the value of the guilt factor. That's always good for something.

Since Viet Nam, I have constantly wondered why God doesn't put an end to wars. Why He does not cure the lame, heal the sick, and prevent these problems that people and children suffer. I really don't get it.

Someone asked once if I knew what "normal" was. I was told a normal person knows that two plus two equals four. A psychotic person knows that two plus two equals five. And a neurotic person knows that two plus two equals four, but it pisses them off.

I have always been a terribly neurotic person. That is my problem and probably has something to do with my mental illness. And that too, pisses me off.

Rachel is currently pregnant. It remains to be seen how this will turn out. Everyone is truly hoping and praying for the best for Rachel and her baby!

She is very upbeat and happy right now. Her thinking is positive about this. The baby was born on September 12, 2022. Rachel seems happy and I began to think this is a good sign. Maybe this will pull her out of her troubles. This was not to be either.

Rachel was excited about being a mother and the way she talked, I believed she would be a good mother. She just seemed up for this.

On the morning of November 14 (Rachel's 21st birthday), they awakened and the baby was not breathing. Ora Lee died. I believe the coroner said it was considered a crib death.

This destroyed Rachel and her boyfriend. Again, I felt completely helpless and could not be there for her support (they live about twelve hours away). After the baby's death, her problems returned and started getting worse again. She also now has severe depression and suicidal thoughts. I do not know where this will end, but I do not believe it will be good.

Over the years, I have tried to reach some conclusions about how all this got started. It is difficult to understand mental issues in a family. This is partly due to the fact that most family members do not want to talk about these things and absolutely do not want to admit that is the case.

Sometimes, no one truly knows the truth, but will say something like, "Charlie was a little strange, but I'm not saying he was crazy." This makes any meaningful research untouchable.

I did discover that I had a great uncle who was born in the early 1900's and his father (my great-grandfather) had him placed in a mental institution in Manteno, Illinois. I don't believe anyone ever knew the truth about why, but there were rumors.

His name was Ralph. He was one of thirteen children, and he was different. One of my mother's sisters told me that Grandpa had Ralph placed there because he was effeminate, and Grandpa did not like that. He wanted his boys strong and tough. I also heard a story that Ralph simply could not cope with life and was considered weak. Another story was that he was always sickly.

Rules were extremely different back then and patients' rights were much worse than they are today. A father can no longer have a child placed in an institution—"just because." However, this is what happened to Ralph from all accounts that I have been able to discover.

At some point, after my great-grandfather died, my great-grandmother asked her other children to try to get Ralph out of the hospital. I understand that it was not easy, but after a couple years of inquiring, they managed to get it done.

If Ralph did not have a problem prior to being placed in Manteno, it became obvious that he did after he was finally released. Ralph did not fit in. It is my belief that he was painfully aware of that.

After two or three years into his release, he asked two of his brothers to take him back to Manteno. It is also my understanding that he made a statement, "That is where my home is."

This, to me, is a very sad comment on what I meant by becoming "institutionalized." And this is what can happen to us when we are not careful.

In this same family, one of the other brothers had some problems once. This was Charlie. He was sitting in the Galesburg Train Station. I do not know why he was there, he just was.

Someone called the police, stating that there is a crazy man sitting at the Depot. Charlie had a habit of gazing at things. Whether it be ants walking across a sidewalk or just staring at nothing (daydreaming). Well, that's what Charlie was doing, and it got him in trouble.

The police summoned a doctor from Mayo Research Institute in Galesburg (later Galesburg Research Hospital). I guess they were not impressed with what Charlie said he was doing.

He was taken to the facility and held for observation for thirty days or thereabouts. They could not find anything actually wrong with my great uncle Charles and had to release him. Charlie was indeed a character… nuts, I do not really think so, but who's to judge?

I did have two cousins that I know of that committed suicide. No one ever had a clue as to what was going on in their lives, what their troubles might have been or why this took place. It is unfortunate.

The End

????

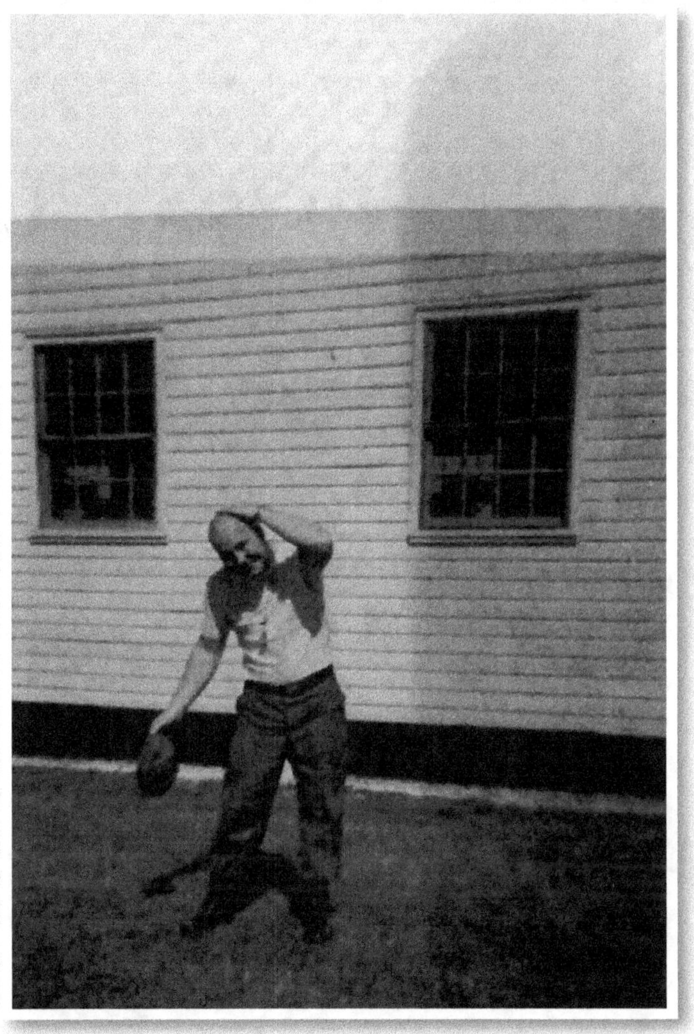

Sep '66 Entered Army

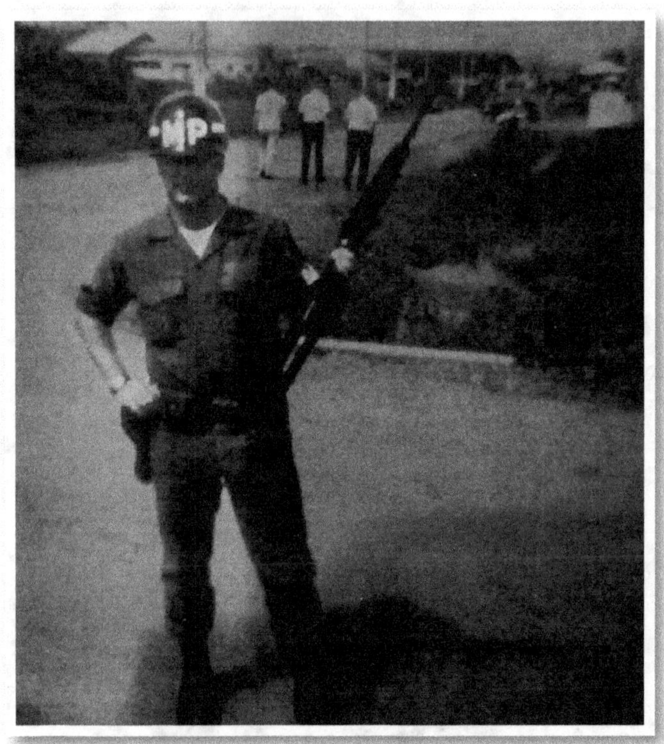

June or July '67 Entered Vietnam

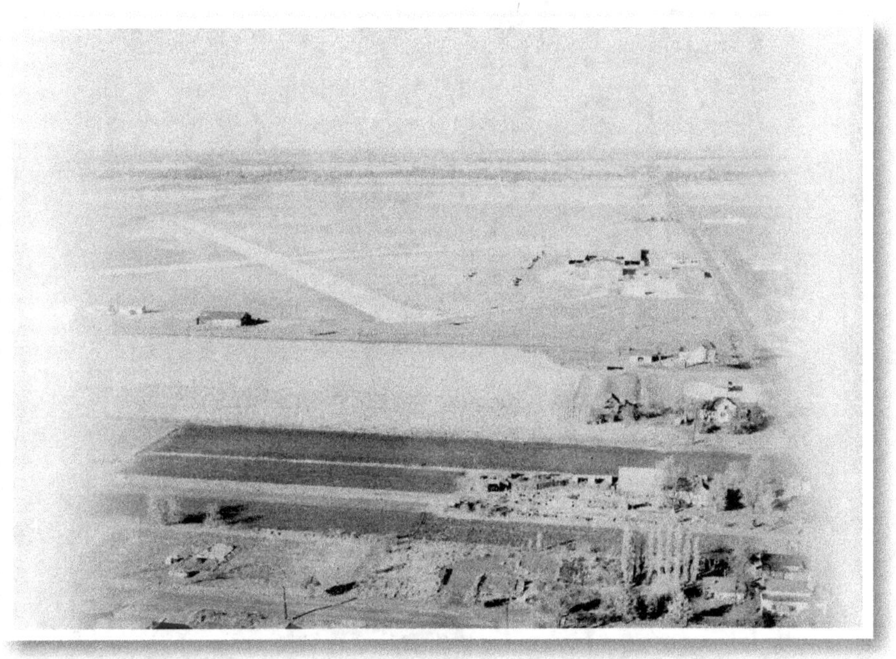

Original Galesburg Airport – Fremont St. and Henderson St.

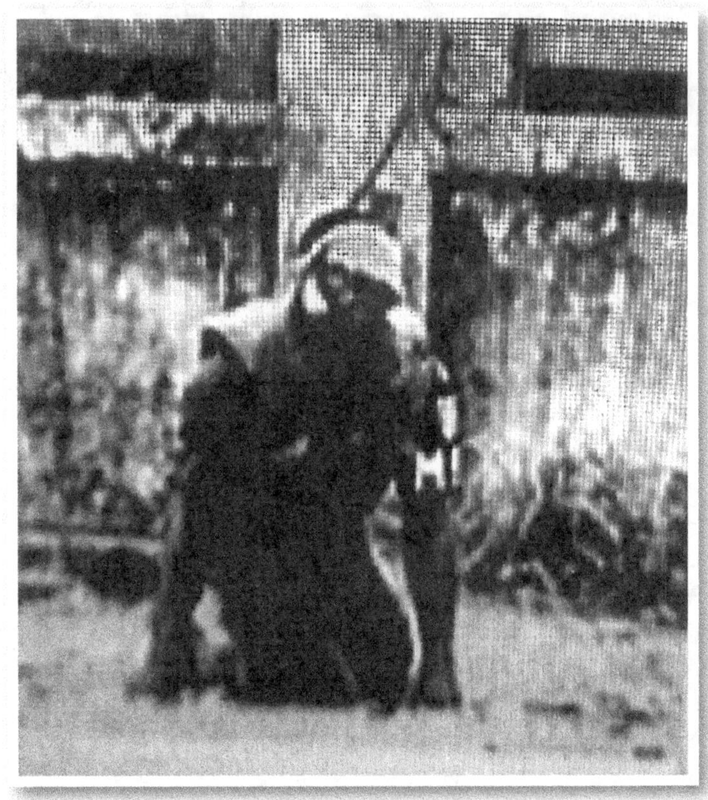

Jefferson at the alley, 1968

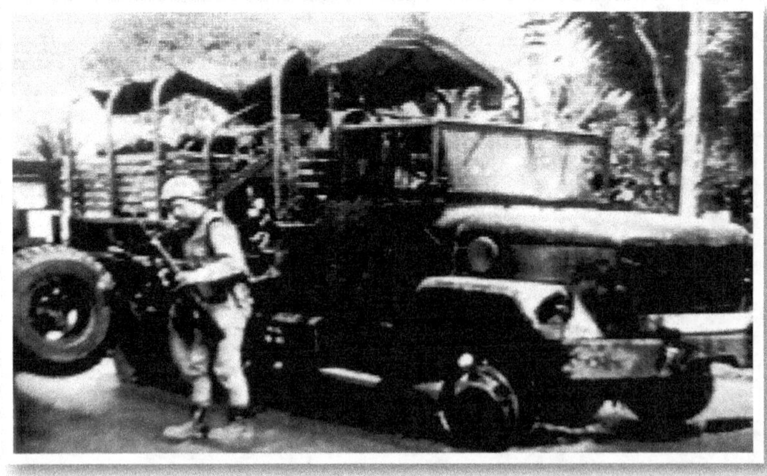

Deuce and a half in the alley, 1968

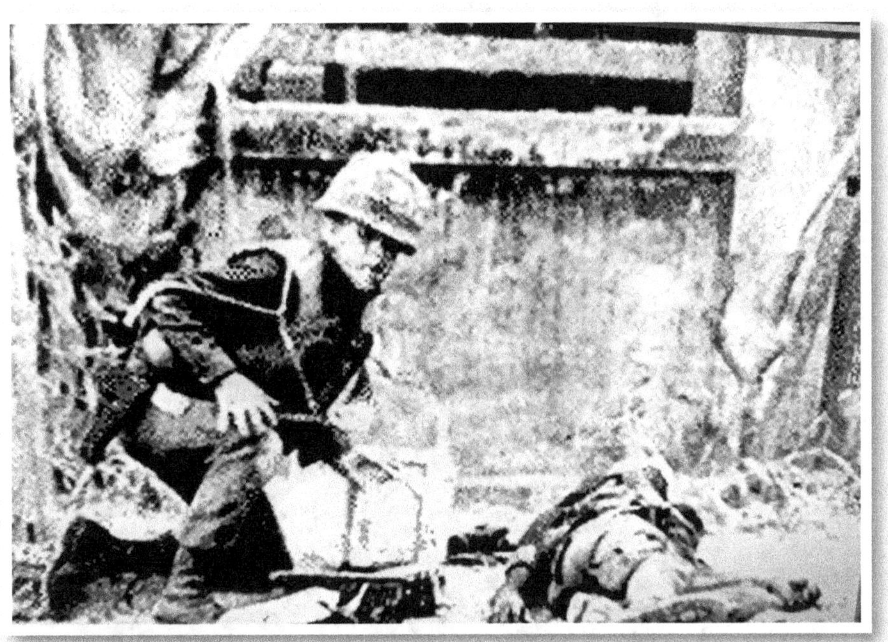

The alley, 1968

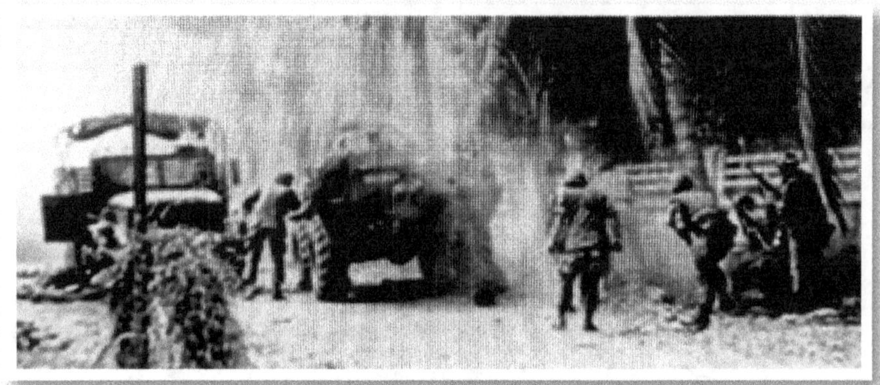

The alley

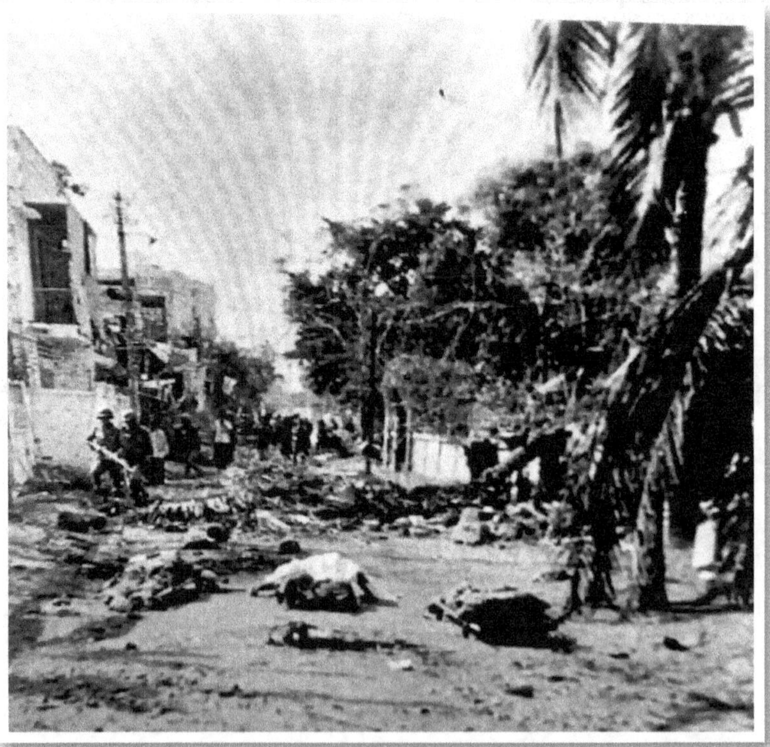

The alley